OXFORD RHEUMATOLOGY

Polymyalgia Rheumatica and Giant Cell Arteritis

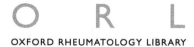

O R L

OXFORD RHEUMATOLOGY LIBRARY

Polymyalgia Rheumatica and Giant Cell Arteritis

Edited by

Bhaskar Dasgupta

Department of Rheumatology, Southend University Hospital, UK

Christian Dejaco

Department of Rheumatology, University of Graz, Austria

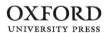

OXFORD
UNIVERSITY PRESS

OXFORD
UNIVERSITY PRESS

Great Clarendon Street, Oxford, OX2 6DP,
United Kingdom

Oxford University Press is a department of the University of Oxford.
It furthers the University's objective of excellence in research, scholarship,
and education by publishing worldwide. Oxford is a registered trade mark of
Oxford University Press in the UK and in certain other countries

First Edition published in 2016

Impression: 1

Published in the United States of America by Oxford University Press
198 Madison Avenue, New York, NY 10016, United States of America

British Library Cataloguing in Publication Data

Data available

Library of Congress Control Number: 2015951525

ISBN 978-0-19-872920-4

Printed in Great Britain by
Clays Ltd, St Ives plc

Foreword

It gives me great pleasure to introduce this Oxford pocketbook on polymyalgia rheumatica and giant cell arteritis (GCA), a publication that arrives not before its time. The conditions account for the majority of long-term steroids prescribed in the community and this book is likely to benefit a readership including general practitioners, hospital specialists, nurses, allied health personnel, patients, and a broader lay audience.

As Chief Executive of a busy NHS Trust, it delights me to note the multidisciplinary, patient-centred focus of a book that attempts to disperse the fog of misconceptions that still shrouds these previously poorly researched illnesses. I see how research and service can come together for the benefit of patients, as exemplified by the fast-track GCA pathway that has shown a cost-effective reduction of sight loss that until today remains the dreaded badge of this disease.

As a person with a lifetime nursing background I felt especially heartened by the chapter on patient and nursing perspectives, which highlights the work being done by patient charities to improve public and professional awareness; and the need to provide close patient support so that sufferers do not feel abandoned at the hour of their need.

While researching this foreword I became aware of Dr Bayard Horton, a distinguished physician from the Mayo Clinic, who originally described temporal arteritis. I note with interest that he was also an inspiring teacher who felt that 'Wonder is the chief ingredient of the investigator. But ... if a man ever expects to do so he must wear his "working shoes" '.

It gives me pride to commend this book, which reflects an international authorship, all stalwarts in their field, but with their working clinical boots firmly strapped on.

Sue Hardy
Chief Executive
Southend University Hospital NHS Foundation Trust

Preface

The twin topics of this book, polymyalgia rheumatica (PMR) and giant cell arteritis (GCA), account for the commonest causes for long-term steroid treatment in the community. PMR is the rheumatic disease subject to the widest variations of clinical practice due to the considerable uncertainty related to diagnosis and outcomes. GCA is a critically ischaemic disease that presents, like PMR, with a broad spectrum of clinical manifestations often complicated by acute ischaemic events including permanent visual loss or stroke.

Early accurate recognition, diagnosis, and adequate treatment of the conditions are thus imperative to prevent loss of independence and to maintain quality of life. Unfortunately these conditions, exclusively occurring in older people, have thus far been deemed 'treatable' unimportant disorders due to a traditionally sanctioned notion of 'unique steroid responsiveness'—despite the absence of any supportive credible evidence for this view. This preconception often becomes a pitfall due to the initial subjective improvement seen in many serious and non-serious conditions in response to high-dose steroid therapy.

Corticosteroids remain as the cornerstone of treatment of PMR and GCA; treatment-related complications are thus a significant burden to patients. The value of steroid-sparing agents is unclear and is being addressed by emerging current and future research. There is an overlap between PMR, GCA, and large-vessel vasculitis (presciently termed as 'polymyalgia arteritica' by Hamrin 60 years ago) and many inflammatory arthritides, connective tissue diseases, and vasculitides have a polymyalgic onset in older people. This makes imaging, with ultrasound and other modalities such as magnetic resonance imaging and positron emission tomography-computed tomography, integral to the management of these conditions.

This pocketbook on PMR and GCA is intended to provide quick and practically relevant information on several aspects of the diseases, particularly on diagnosis and management. Ultimately, the aim of this book is to improve patient care.

The intended audience is the rheumatologist, general practitioner, and other professionals for caring patients with PMR and GCA.

There have been recent advances in these areas. The provisional European League Against Rheumatism/American College of Rheumatology (EULAR/ACR) PMR classification criteria have been published, EULAR/ACR PMR guidelines are awaiting publication, and national international guidelines are being disseminated for GCA. The fast-track GCA pathway, shown to reduce sight loss, is gaining ground as the standard of care. PMRGCAuk, a charity designated exclusively for these conditions, is working tirelessly to increase public and professional awareness and offer support to patients.

This pocketbook, written by international experts, highlights current concepts of pathogenesis as well as recent advances of diagnostic and therapeutic approaches. Ongoing research aims at the identification of new biomarkers and corticosteroid-sparing medications, which should improve the long-term outcome of PMR and GCA patients. Each chapter is complemented with 'key points' boxes, highlighting the most relevant information for clinical practice. Practical flowcharts (e.g. on diagnostic work-up and treatment) are also provided.

We are most grateful to Oxford University Press and our many international colleagues who have worked tirelessly to bring this unique publication effort to fruition.

Contents

Abbreviations   *xi*
Contributors   *xiii*

Part 1 Epidemiology, pathogenesis, and clinical presentation

1 Definition and epidemiology   **3**
   Miguel A. González-Gay, Trinitario Pina, and Ricardo Blanco

2 Aetiology and pathogenesis   **11**
   Georgina Espígol-Frigolé, Ester Planas-Rigol, Marc Corbera-Bellalta,
   Nekane Terrades-García, Marco A. Alba, Sergio Prieto-González,
   José Hernández-Rodríguez, Bhaskar Dasgupta, and Maria C. Cid

3 Clinical presentation and classification criteria
   for polymyalgia rheumatica   **25**
   Wiliam Docken, Eric L. Matteson, and Bhaskar Dasgupta

4 Clinical manifestations of giant cell arteritis   **33**
   Carlo Salvarani and Nicolò Pipitone

Part 2 Diagnostic work-up

5 Laboratory findings   **43**
   Nicolò Pipitone

6 Ultrasound   **49**
   Wolfgang A. Schmidt

7 Temporal artery biopsy   **59**
   Francesco Muratore and Nicolò Pipitone

8 Positron emission tomography and magnetic resonance imaging   **63**
   Daniel E. Blockmans

9 Differential diagnosis   **73**
   Dario Camellino and Marco A. Cimmino

Part 3 Guidelines for treatment

10 Glucocorticoids **81**
Frank Buttgereit

11 Role of steroid-sparing agents **89**
Christian Dejaco

12 Treatment of a relapse and approach to difficult-to-treat patients **97**
Bhaskar Dasgupta

13 Management of sight loss and other disease-
and treatment-related complications **103**
Pravin Patil, Niral Karia, and Bhaskar Dasgupta

Part 4 Outcomes, prognosis, socioeconomic implications, primary care, and patient perspectives

14 Determination of disease activity and outcomes **119**
Christian Dejaco

15 Prognosis and duration of therapy **125**
Sarah L. Mackie

16 Primary care **133**
Toby Helliwell, Samantha L. Hider, and Christian D. Mallen

17 Socioeconomic implications **139**
Matthew J. Koster, Eric L. Matteson, and Cynthia S. Crowson

18 Patient education **145**
Kate Gilbert

Index *151*

Abbreviations

ACPA	anticyclic citrullinated peptide antibody
ACR	American College of Rheumatology
ANA	antinuclear antibody
ANCA	antineutrophil cytoplasmic antibody
BSR	British Society for Rheumatology
CDS	colour duplex sonography
cGCR	cytosolic glucocorticoid receptor
CI	confidence interval
CPPD	calcium pyrophosphate deposition disease
CRP	C-reactive protein
DMARD	disease-modifying antirheumatic drug
EORA	elderly-onset rheumatoid arthritis
EULAR	European League Against Rheumatism
FDG	fluorodeoxyglucose
GC	glucocorticoid
GCA	giant cell arteritis
GP	general practitioner
GVK	gevokizumab
HLA	human leucocyte antigen
IFN	interferon
IL	interleukin
LVV	large-vessel vasculitis
MHC	major histocompatibility complex
MMP	matrix metalloprotease
MPA	microscopic polyangiitis *or* methylprednisolone
MRA	magnetic resonance angiography
MTX	methotrexate
NSAID	non-steroidal anti-inflammatory drug
OR	odds ratio
PCR	polymyalgia rheumatica
PET	positron emission tomography
PM	polymyositis
PMRGCAuk	Polymyalgia Rheumatica and Giant Cell Arteritis UK

RA	rheumatoid arthritis
RCT	randomized controlled trial
TAB	temporal artery biopsy
TAK	Takayasu's arteritis
TCZ	tocilizumab
TGF	transforming growth factor
Th	T helper
TNFa	tumour necrosis factor alpha
VEGF	vascular endothelial growth factor

Contributors

Marco A. Alba

Department of Autoimmune Diseases, Hospital Clínic, University of Barcelona, Institut d'Investigacions Biomèdiques August Pi I Sunyer (IDIBAPS), Barcelona, Spain

Ricardo Blanco

Rheumatology Section, Hospital Universitario Marques de Valdecilla, Santander, Spain

Daniel E. Blockmans

University Hospital Gasthuisberg, Department of General Internal Medicine, Leuven, Belgium

Frank Buttgereit

Department of Rheumatology and Clinical Immunology, Charité University Hospital, Humboldt University, Berlin, Germany

Dario Camellino

Clinical Rheumatology, University of Genoa, Genoa, Italy

Maria C. Cid

Department of Autoimmune Diseases, Hospital Clínic, University of Barcelona, Institut d'Investigacions Biomèdiques August Pi I Sunyer (IDIBAPS), Barcelona, Spain

Marco A. Cimmino

Clinical Rheumatology, University of Genoa, Genoa, Italy

Marc Corbera-Bellalta

Department of Autoimmune Diseases, Hospital Clínic, University of Barcelona, Institut d'Investigacions Biomèdiques August Pi I Sunyer (IDIBAPS), Barcelona, Spain

Cynthia S. Crowson

Mayo Clinic, Rochester, MN, USA

Bhaskar Dasgupta

Department of Rheumatology, Southend University Hospital, Westcliff-on-Sea, UK

Christian Dejaco

Division of Rheumatology and Immunology, Medical University of Graz, Graz, Austria

Wiliam Docken

Brigham and Women's Hospital, Boston, MA, USA

Georgina Espígol-Frigolé

Department of Autoimmune Diseases, Hospital Clínic, University of Barcelona, Institut d'Investigacions Biomèdiques August Pi I Sunyer (IDIBAPS), Barcelona, Spain

Kate Gilbert

Polymyalgia Rheumatica and Giant Cell Arteritis UK (PMRGCAuk), UK

Miguel A. González-Gay

Rheumatology Section, Hospital Universitario Marques de Valdecilla, Santander, Spain

Toby Helliwell

Institute for Primary Care and Health Sciences, Keele University, Keele, UK

José Hernández-Rodríguez

Department of Autoimmune Diseases, Hospital Clínic, University of Barcelona, Institut d'Investigacions Biomèdiques August Pi I Sunyer (IDIBAPS), Barcelona, Spain

Samantha L. Hider

Institute for Primary Care and Health Sciences, Keele University, Keele, UK

Niral Karia

Department of Ophthalmology, Southend University Hospital, Westcliff-on-Sea, UK

Matthew J. Koster

Mayo Clinic, Rochester, MN, USA

Sarah L. Mackie

Leeds Institute of Rheumatic and Musculoskeletal Medicine, University of Leeds, Leeds, UK

Christian D. Mallen

Institute for Primary Care and Health Sciences, Keele University, Keele, UK

Eric L. Matteson

Rheumatology Division, Mayo Clinic, Rochester, MN, USA

Francesco Muratore

Unit of Rheumatology, Arcispedale Santa Maria Nuova – IRCCS, Reggio Emilia, Italy

Pravin Patil

Aditya Birla Hospital, Mumbai, India

Trinitario Pina

Rheumatology Section, Hospital Universitario Marques de Valdecilla, Santander, Spain

Nicolò Pipitone

Unit of Rheumatology, Arcispedale Santa Maria Nuova – IRCCS, Reggio Emilia, Italy

Ester Planas-Rigol

Department of Autoimmune Diseases, Hospital Clínic, University of Barcelona, Institut d'Investigacions Biomèdiques August Pi I Sunyer (IDIBAPS), Barcelona, Spain

Sergio Prieto-González

Department of Autoimmune Diseases, Hospital Clínic, University of Barcelona, Institut d'Investigacions Biomèdiques August Pi I Sunyer (IDIBAPS), Barcelona, Spain

Carlo Salvarani

Unit of Rheumatology, Arcispedale Santa Maria Nuova – IRCCS, Reggio Emilia, Italy

Wolfgang A. Schmidt

Immanuel Krankenhaus Berlin, Medical Centre for Rheumatology Berlin-Buch, Berlin, Germany

Nekane Terrades-García

Department of Autoimmune Diseases, Hospital Clínic, University of Barcelona, Institut d'Investigacions Biomèdiques August Pi I Sunyer (IDIBAPS), Barcelona, Spain

Part 1

Epidemiology, pathogenesis, and clinical presentation

1	Definition and epidemiology	**3**
2	Aetiology and pathogenesis	**11**
3	Clinical presentation and classification criteria for polymyalgia rheumatica	**25**
4	Clinical manifestations of giant cell arteritis	**33**

Chapter 1

Definition and epidemiology

Miguel A. González-Gay, Trinitario Pina, and Ricardo Blanco

Key points

- Polymyalgia rheumatica (PMR) and giant cell arteritis (GCA) are common, overlapping conditions that almost exclusively occur in people older than 50 years of age.
- Environmental factors and infectious agents have been proposed to be involved in the pathogenesis of PMR and GCA.
- GCA is strongly associated with *HLA-DRB1*04* alleles.

1.1 Definition

PMR is characterized by pain and stiffness involving the shoulder girdle, proximal aspects of the arms, the neck, and the pelvic girdle. PMR is associated with morning stiffness and, as observed in GCA, it occurs more commonly in individuals aged 50 years and older (1,2). In patients with PMR, magnetic resonance imaging and ultrasonography often show inflammation of subacromial subdeltoid bursae, synovitis of the glenohumeral joints, tenosynovitis of the long head of biceps, as well as trochanteric, iliopsoas, ischiogluteal, and interspinous bursitis (3–5).

GCA, also called temporal arteritis, is a vasculitis that affects large and middle-sized blood vessels with predominant involvement of cranial arteries derived from the carotid artery, in individuals older than 50 years of age (1). Although the typical manifestations of GCA are the result of the involvement of the external carotid artery, the most feared manifestation is blindness due to anterior ischaemic optic neuropathy that is usually the result of the vasculitic damage of the posterior ciliary arteries branches from the internal carotid artery (6). Moreover, aortic involvement in GCA may be found in one-half to two-thirds of patients using fluorodeoxyglucose positron emission tomography and computed tomography (7). Patients with large-vessel GCA primarily involving the upper extremities often do not have the typical cranial features of GCA (8).

1.2 Epidemiology

1.2.1 General considerations

PMR and GCA are overlapping conditions (9) with approximately 40–60% of individuals with GCA exhibiting polymyalgic manifestations. In 10–20% of patients, PMR may be the presenting symptom of GCA (9).

PMR is more common than GCA (1,2). PMR may present as an isolated entity (10) or be the presenting feature in patients who later develop typical cranial manifestations of GCA. Population-based studies have shown the presence of 'silent' biopsy-proven GCA in 9–21% of the patients presenting with PMR features (3). Also, PMR manifestations are observed in up to 40–50% of patients with biopsy-proven GCA (11).

1.2.2 Incidence of GCA and PMR

Both PMR and GCA are commoner in Western countries, in particular in white individuals of Scandinavian background (1). CGA is uncommon in Asian populations. The prevalence of patients aged 50 and older in Japan was 1.47/100,000 compared with 200 and 60 cases/100,000 people in the United States and Spain, respectively (12). A north–south gradient in the incidence of GCA was seen in Europe with high rates in Sweden and Norway (generally more than 20 new cases of GCA/100,000 individuals aged 50 and older per year) and lower incidence in Southern Europe (annual incidence rate of 10 cases/100,000 people aged 50 years and older in northwestern Spain) (1). PMR and GCA are seen more often in women, in particular in the 70–79-year-old age group (1, 13). Incidence of GCA and PMR is lower in Hispanic, Asian, and African American populations (1). A recent study focusing on the epidemiology of GCA in Mexican Mestizos confirmed that GCA is uncommon in Latin America (14). In Olmsted County, Minnesota, USA, incidence rates have remained stable since 1970 (15).

Incidence rates of GCA in different parts of the world are summarized in Table 1.1.

As reported for GCA, the incidence of PMR has been found to be higher in individuals of Scandinavian background (16–18). In this regard, the annual incidence rate of PMR in Ribe County, Denmark, over the period 1982–1985 was 68.3/100,000 for the population aged 50 years or older (16). Likewise, the incidence of PMR in Göteborg, Sweden, between 1985 and 1987 for the population aged 50 years or over was 50/100,000 (17). In Olmsted County, Minnesota, USA, where the population has a strong Scandinavian background, the annual incidence rate of PMR for individuals aged 50 years or older between 1970 and 1999 was 58.7/100,000 (18). In contrast, as described for GCA, the annual incidence of PMR is lower in Southern European countries. In this regard, the annual incidence rate of PMR in Reggio Emilia, Italy, over the period 1980–1988 for the population aged 50 years or older was 12.7/100,000 (19). Incidence of PMR in different parts of the world is shown in Table 1.2.

1.2.3 Influence of environmental factors and infectious agents

Environmental factors and infectious agents have been proposed to play a role in the pathogenesis of PMR and GCA (20). Fluctuations in the incidence of PMR and GCA in different regions of Denmark contemporaneous with *Mycoplasma pneumonia*, parvovirus B19, and *Chlamydia pneumoniae* epidemics have been reported (17). The reinfection with human parainfluenza virus type 1 was also associated with the onset of GCA, particularly in biopsy-proven patients (21).

A regular epidemic-like cyclical pattern in incidence rates of GCA with peaks in the incidence every 7 years over a 42-year period was found in Olmsted County,

Table 1.1 Incidence of giant cell arteritis		
Location	Years of study	Incidence/10^{5a}
Scandinavian countries:		
Skane County, Sweden	1997–2010	14.1[b]
Vest Agder County, Norway	1992–1996	29.1[b]
Aust Agder, Norway	1987–1994	29.0
Iceland	1984–1990	27.0
Ribe County, Denmark	1982–1985	23.3
Göteborg, Sweden	1976–1995	22.2[b]
Olmsted County, MN, USA (Scandinavian background)	2000–2009	19.8
	1950–1999	18.8
	1950–1991	17.8
	1950–1985	17.0
Lugo, Spain	1981–1998	10.2
	1981–2005	10.1[b]
Israel	1980–1991	10.2
	1980–2004	9.5[b]
Loire-Atlantique, France	1970–1979	9.4
Reggio Emilia, Italy	1980–1988	6.9

[a] For population aged 50 years or older.

[b] Including only biopsy-proven GCA patients.

Gonzalez-Gay MA, Vazquez-Rodriguez TR, Lopez-Diaz MJ, et al. Epidemiology of giant cell arteritis and polymyalgia rheumatica. Arthritis & Rheumatism, 61: 1454–1461, 2009, Wiley. Chandran A, Udayakumar P, Crowson C, Warrington K, Matteson E. The incidence of giant cell arteritis in Olmsted County, Minnesota, over a 60-year period 1950–2009. Scand J Rheumatol 2015; 44(3):215–18. Adapted by permission from BMJ Publishing Group Limited. Mohammad AJ, Nilsson JA, Jacobsson LT, Merkel PA, Turesson C., Ann Rheum Dis, 74, 6, 993–997, 2015 copyright.

Minnesota, USA (22). Cyclic fluctuations of age-adjusted GCA incidence with three distinctive peaks, 8–10 years apart, were also found in Jerusalem, Israel, over the period 1980–2004 (23). Some investigators have also reported a seasonal distribution of GCA.

Regrettably, several studies have failed to confirm any association between the presence of parvovirus B19, Chlamydia pneumoniae, or human herpes virus DNA in temporal artery biopsy specimens and the histological evidence of biopsy-proven GCA (24–26). The contribution of varicella zoster virus to development of GCA remains to be an issue of speculation and controversy (27,28).

1.2.4 Implication of genetic factors

A genetic component, in particular in patients with biopsy-proven GCA, has been reported (29). A strong association between GCA and HLA-DRB1*04 alleles of the human leucocyte antigen (HLA) region has been described in most studies (30) (Table 1.3). However, this was not the case for series dealing with isolated PMR (29). Additional genetic associations with GCA, such as the classical functional PTPN22 (protein tyrosine

Table 1.2 Incidence of polymyalgia rheumatica

Location	Years of study	Incidence rate/10[5a]
Ribe County, Denmark	1982–1985	68.3
Olmsted County, MN, USA	1970–1991	52.5
Göteborg, Sweden	1985–1987	50.0[b]
Denmark (different areas)	1982–1984	41.3
Lugo, Spain (total)	1987–1996	18.7
Lugo, Spain (isolated)	1987–1996	13.5[c]
Reggio Emilia, Italy	1980–1988	12.7

[a] For population aged 50 years or older.

[b] Including only patients with polymyalgia rheumatica and no histological evidence of GCA.

[c] Including only patients with isolated ('pure') PMR.

Reproduced from Gonzalez-Gay MA, Vazquez-Rodriguez TR, Lopez-Diaz MJ, et al. Epidemiology of giant cell arteritis and polymyalgia rheumatic, *Arthritis & Rheumatism*, 61: 1454–1461, 2009, with permission from Wiley.

phosphatase, non-receptor type 22 (lymphoid)) allele rs2476601 (R620W) A, have recently been described (31). The use of the new technologies available for the genetic studies, such as genome-wide association studies, will help to disclose the genetic component of these conditions (32).

1.2.5 Influence of classic cardiovascular risk factors

A strong association between smoking and previous atheromatous disease in women with GCA was proposed (33). The presence of atherosclerosis risk factors at the time of diagnosis of GCA, in particular hypertension, has also been associated with an increased risk of severe ischaemic complications (34).

Table 1.3 Main genetic studies on *HLA-DRB1*04* allele association in giant cell arteritis

Year of publication	Location	HLA-DRB1*04 association	Cohort analysed (case–control)	P-value
1992	Rochester, MN, USA[a]	Yes	42/63	0.03
1994	Rochester, MN, USA[a]	Yes	52/72	0.0001
1998	Toulouse (France)	Yes	41/384	<0.001
1998	Montpellier (France)	Yes	42/1609	0.0005
1998	Lugo (Spain)	Yes	53/145	<0.05
1999	Reggio Emilia (Italy)	No	39/250	NS
2002	Copenhagen (Denmark)	Yes	65/193	0.01

[a] Scandinavian descent.

Reproduced from Salvarani C, Farnetti E, Casali B, et al. Detection of parvovirus B19 DNA by polymerase chain reaction in giant cell arteritis: a case-control study, *Arthritis & Rheumatism*, 46: 3099–3101, 2002, with permission from Wiley.

1.2.6 **Outcome**

Most population-based studies have not shown an increased incidence of cancer in GCA (35, 36). Nevertheless, a recent UK study of the GPRD database suggested an increased risk of cancer diagnosis within the first 6 months after a PMR diagnosis (37). A study in 2013 suggests that the use of statins may reduce the risk of GCA (38). Another report from 2014 suggests that cardiovascular disease may be increased in patients with GCA (39). However, most long-term survival studies have shown no excess mortality in patients with PMR and GCA (19, 20, 40–42), although one Swedish study has reported increased early mortality (43). This may be particularly true in the subgroup with irreversible sight loss. Early cardiovascular events have also been reported recently in GCA (39).

1.3 **Conclusion**

PMR and GCA are common and often overlapping conditions in people older than 50 years in Western countries. Peaks in the incidence and a cyclic pattern observed in some studies suggest that infectious agents may play a role in the pathogenesis of both diseases.

References

1. Gonzalez-Gay MA, Vazquez-Rodriguez TR, Lopez-Diaz MJ, et al. Epidemiology of giant cell arteritis and polymyalgia rheumatica. *Arthritis Rheum* 2009; 61:1454–61.

2. Salvarani C, Cantini F, Hunder GG. Polymyalgia rheumatica and giant-cell arteritis. *Lancet* 2008, 372:234–45.

3. Salvarani C, Cantini F, Olivieri I, et al. Proximal bursitis in active polymyalgia rheumatica. *Ann Intern Med* 1997; 127:27–31.

4. Cantini F, Niccoli L, Nannini C, et al. Inflammatory changes of hip synovial structures in polymyalgia rheumatica. *Clin Exp Rheumatol* 2005; 23:462–8.

5. Salvarani C, Barozzi L, Cantini F, et al. Cervical interspinous bursitis in active polymyalgia rheumatica. *Ann Rheum Dis* 2008; 67:758–61.

6. González-Gay MA, García-Porrúa C, Llorca J, et al. Visual manifestations of giant cell arteritis. Trends and clinical spectrum in 161 patients. *Medicine (Baltimore)* 2000; 79:283–92.

7. Muratore F, Pazzola G, Pipitone N, et al. Large-vessel involvement in giant cell arteritis and polymyalgia rheumatica. *Clin Exp Rheumatol* 2014; 32(3 Suppl 82): S106–S11.

8. Muratore F, Kermani TA, Crowson CS, et al. Large-vessel giant cell arteritis: a cohort study. *Rheumatology (Oxford)* 2015; 54(3):463–70.

9. Gonzalez-Gay MA. Giant cell arteritis and polymyalgia rheumatica: two different but often overlapping conditions. *Semin Arthritis Rheum* 2004; 33:289–93.

10. Gonzalez-Gay MA, Garcia-Porrua C, Vazquez-Caruncho M. Polymyalgia rheumatica in biopsy proven giant cell arteritis does not constitute a different subset but differs from isolated polymyalgia rheumatica. *J Rheumatol* 1998; 25:1750–5.

11. Gonzalez-Gay MA, Barros S, Lopez-Diaz MJ, et al. Giant cell arteritis: disease patterns of clinical presentation in a series of 240 patients. *Medicine (Baltimore)* 2005; 84:269–76.

12. Kobayashi S, Fujimoto S. Epidemiology of vasculitides: differences between Japan, Europe and North America. *Clin Exp Nephrol* 2013; 17:611–14.

13. Petri H, Nevitt A, Sarsour K, et al. Incidence of giant cell arteritis and characteristics of patients: data-driven analysis of comorbidities. *Arthritis Care Res (Hoboken)* 2015; 67(3):390–5.

14. Alba MA, Mena-Madrazo JA, Reyes E, et al. Giant cell arteritis in Mexican patients. J Clin Rheumatol 2012; 18:1–7.

15. Chandran A, Udayakumar P, Crowson C, et al. The incidence of giant cell arteritis in Olmsted County, Minnesota, over a 60-year period 1950–2009. Scand J Rheumatol 2015; 44(3):215–18.

16. Boesen P, Sorensen SF. Giant cell arteritis, temporal arteritis, and polymyalgia rheumatica in a Danish county: a prospective investigation, 1982–1985. Arthritis Rheum 1987; 30:294–9.

17. Elling P, Olsson AT, Elling H. Synchronous variations of the incidence of temporal arteritis and polymyalgia rheumatica in different regions of Denmark; association with epidemics of Mycoplasma pneumoniae infection. J Rheumatol 1996; 23:112–19.

18. Doran MF, Crowson CS, O'Fallon WM, et al. Trends in the incidence of polymyalgia rheumatic over a 30 year period in Olmsted County, Minnesota, USA. J Rheumatol 2002; 29:1694–7.

19. González-Gay MA, García-Porrúa C, Vázquez-Caruncho M, et al. The spectrum of polymyalgia rheumatica in northwestern Spain: incidence and analysis of variables associated with relapse in a 10 year study. J Rheumatol 1999; 26:1326–32.

20. Gonzalez-Gay MA, Garcia-Porrua C. Epidemiology of the vasculitides. Rheum Dis Clin North Am 2001; 27:729–49.

21. Duhaut P, Bosshard S, Calvet A, et al. Giant cell arteritis, polymyalgia rheumatica, and viral hypotheses: a multicenter, prospective case-control study. Groupe de Recherche sur l'Arterite a Cellules Geantes. J Rheumatol 1999; 26:361–9.

22. Salvarani C, Gabriel SE, O'Fallon WM, et al. The incidence of giant cell arteritis in Olmsted County, Minnesota: apparent fluctuations in a cyclic pattern. Ann Intern Med 1995; 123:192–4.

23. Bas-Lando M, Breuer GS, Berkun Y, et al. The incidence of giant cell arteritis in Jerusalem over a 25-year period: annual and seasonal fluctuations. Clin Exp Rheumatol 2007; 25(1 Suppl 44):S15–17.

24. Regan MJ, Wood BJ, Hsieh YH, et al. Temporal arteritis and Chlamydia pneumoniae: failure to detect the organism by polymerase chain reaction in ninety cases and ninety controls. Arthritis Rheum 2002; 46:1056–60.

25. Salvarani C, Farnetti E, Casali B, et al. Detection of parvovirus B19 DNA by polymerase chain reaction in giant cell arteritis: a case–control study. Arthritis Rheum 2002; 46:3099–101.

26. Rodriguez-Pla A, Bosch-Gil JA, Echevarria-Mayo JE, et al. No detection of parvovirus B19 or herpesvirus DNA in giant cell arteritis. J Clin Virol 2004; 31:11–15.

27. Mitchell BM, Font RL. Detection of varicella zoster virus DNA in some patients with giant cell arteritis. Invest Ophthalmol Vis Sci 2001; 42:2572–7.

28. Gilden D, White T, Khmeleva N, et al. Prevalence and distribution of VZV in temporal arteries of patients with giant cell arteritis. Neurology 2015; 84(19):1948–55.

29. González-Gay MA, Amoli MM, Garcia-Porrua C, et al. Genetic markers of disease susceptibility and severity in giant cell arteritis and polymyalgia rheumatica. Semin Arthritis Rheum 2003; 33:38–48.

30. Carmona FD, González-Gay MA, Martín J. Genetic component of giant cell arteritis. Rheumatology (Oxford) 2014; 53:6–18.

31. Serrano A, Márquez A, Mackie SL, et al. Identification of the PTPN22 functional variant R620W as susceptibility genetic factor for giant cell arteritis. Ann Rheum Dis 2013; 72:1882–6.

32. Carmona FD, Martín J, González-Gay MA. Genetics of vasculitis. Curr Opin Rheumatol 2015; 27:10–17.

33. Duhaut P, Pinede L, Demolombe-Rague S, et al. Giant cell arteritis and cardiovascular risk factors. A multicenter, prospective case-control study. Arthritis Rheum 1998; 41:1960–5.

34. Gonzalez-Gay MA, Piñeiro A, Gomez-Gigirey A, et al. Influence of traditional risk factors of atherosclerosis in the development of severe ischemic complications in giant cell arteritis. Medicine (Baltimore) 2004; 83:342–7.

35. Gonzalez-Gay MA, Lopez-Diaz MJ, Martinez-Lado L, et al. Cancer in biopsy-proven giant cell arteritis. A population-based study. Semin Arthritis Rheum 2007; 37:156–63.

36. Kermani TA, Schäfer VS, Crowson CS, et al. Malignancy risk in patients with giant cell arteritis: a population-based cohort study. Arthritis Care Res (Hoboken) 2010; 62:149–54.

37. Muller S, Hider SL, Belcher J, et al. Is cancer associated with polymyalgia rheumatica? A cohort study in the General Practice Research Database. Ann Rheum Dis 2014; 73:1769–73.

38. Schmidt J, Kermani TA, Muratore F, et al. Statin use in giant cell arteritis: a retrospective study. J Rheumatol 2013; 40:910–15.

39. Tomasson G, Peloquin C, Mohammad A, et al. Risk for cardiovascular disease early and late after a diagnosis of giant-cell arteritis: a cohort study. Ann Intern Med 2014; 160:73–80.

40. Matteson EL, Gold KN, Bloch DA, et al. Long-term survival of patients with giant cell arteritis in the American College of Rheumatology giant cell arteritis classification criteria cohort. Am J Med 1996; 100:193–6.

41. Gonzalez-Gay MA, Blanco R, Abraira V, et al. Giant cell arteritis in Lugo, Spain, is associated with low longterm mortality. J Rheumatol 1997; 24:2171–6.

42. Gran JT, Myklebust G, Wilsgaard T, et al. Survival in polymyalgia rheumatica and temporal arteritis: a study of 398 cases and matched population controls. Rheumatology (Oxford) 2001; 40:1238–42.

43. Mohammad AJ, Nilsson JA, Jacobsson LT, et al. Incidence and mortality rates of biopsy-proven giant cell arteritis in southern Sweden. Ann Rheum Dis 2015; 74(6):993–7.

Chapter 2

Aetiology and pathogenesis

Georgina Espígol-Frigolé, Ester Planas-Rigol, Marc Corbera-Bellalta,
Nekane Terrades-García, Marco A. Alba, Sergio Prieto-González,
José Hernández-Rodríguez, Bhaskar Dasgupta,* and Maria C. Cid*

> **Key points**
>
> - Genetic background plays a significant role in the pathogenesis of polymyalgia rheumatica (PMR) and giant cell arteritis (GCA).
> - Both T-helper (Th)1- and Th17-mediated immune responses contribute to the development of vascular inflammation in GCA. Activated macrophages participate in amplification cascades and vascular injury. Mechanisms of synovial inflammation in PMR are less understood.
> - Vascular remodelling in response to inflammation leads to vascular occlusion and ischaemic complications in GCA.

2.1 Introduction

PMR and GCA are pathogenetically closely related conditions. While PMR is a synovial inflammatory disease, mainly involving proximal joints and periarticular structures, GCA is a granulomatous vasculitis involving large and medium-sized vessels (Figure 2.1) (1). PMR shares many epidemiological and demographic characteristics with GCA and it is actually a prominent part of the clinical picture in about 50% of patients with GCA. In these patients, PMR may precede, be coincident, or develop after the appearance of vascular symptoms (2). PMR may also exist as a distinct entity in patients with no evidence of vascular inflammation and may be part of the picture of other rheumatic diseases including late-onset rheumatoid arthritis and spondyloarthropathies.

The pathogenesis of PMR and GCA is only partially understood due to the limited availability of functional models where the participation of particular pathways can be mechanistically investigated. The widespread performance of temporal artery biopsies for the diagnosis of GCA has provided valuable tissue not only for diagnostic purposes but also for immunopathology studies. Vascular inflammation and remodelling in GCA has been more thoroughly investigated than synovial inflammation in PMR since PMR patients are not routinely subjected to arthroscopic biopsies. The current pathogenesis model is essentially based on the identification of particular cell populations

---

* Shared senior authorship.

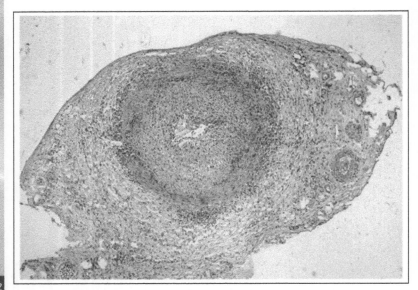

Figure 2.1 (See colour plate section). Temporal artery biopsy from a patient with GCA disclosing typical transmural mononuclear cell infiltration, internal elastic lamina breakdown, and intimal hyperplasia. Haematoxylin–eosin staining.

and subsets in involved tissues and/or peripheral blood, the expression of markers of activation and differentiation, as well as the production of certain inflammatory mediators in inflammatory lesions. For the interpretation of these findings, basic principles of immunology including the role of infiltrating cells and their products are extrapolated, and correlations of histopathological features with clinical phenotypes and disease outcomes are made (3, 4). However, further work is required to confirm our assumptions regarding GCA pathogenesis.

2.2 Predisposing factors

Epidemiological studies strongly indicate that genetic background, senescence, and gender contribute to the pathogenesis of GCA and PMR (5). The role of ageing and sex remain virtually unexplored in PMR or GCA. Recently, senescent T cells (CD4+ CD28−) have been identified in GCA lesions and are increased in peripheral blood from patients with several chronic inflammatory conditions, including GCA and PMR (6). Some of these cells express NKG2D receptors and their ligation induces production of interferon gamma (IFNγ) and tumour necrosis factor alpha (TNFα), which are relevant cytokines in GCA. The pathogenic and functional relevance of these cells in PMR and GCA needs further investigation.

Genetic predisposition to develop GCA has been suspected for a long time because of the strong predominance of GCA among white people, particularly those with Northern European ancestry, and the occasionally observed familiar clustering (5, 7).

Over the years, several studies have identified genetic variants associated with increased risk for PMR or GCA supporting the suspected genetic background for these diseases (reviewed in reference 8). Polymorphisms in a variety of genes encoding for molecules involved in immune and inflammatory responses (i.e. class II major histocompatibility complex (MHC), PTPN22, NOS2, and vascular endothelial growth factor (VEGF)) have been associated with an increased susceptibility to GCA (8–10).

GCA has been repeatedly found to be associated with MHC variants, particularly with class II human leucocyte antigen (HLA) alleles of HLA-DRB1*04 (generally HLA-DRB1*04:01, but also HLA-DRB1*04:04) (8). The association of these alleles with PMR is less coherent, probably because a variety of processes may present as PMR resulting in unavoidable uncertainty surrounding PMR diagnosis (8, 11). A large-scale genetic study based on international multicentre collaboration has recently confirmed that the strongest association of GCA occurs with variants in MHC class II and that the derived risk amino acids are located in the antigen-binding pocket of the HLA molecule (12). This finding reinforces the concept that GCA is an antigen-driven disease.

2.3 Initial events: T-cell activation and functional differentiation

The nature of the triggering agent(s) has not been consistently identified. Various microbe and viral sequences have been detected in temporal artery lesions but no convincing causal relationship with a particular microorganism or virus has been identified (13). Both innate and adaptive mechanisms seem to play a role in GCA (4). Dendritic cells can be identified in lesions (14) and can be activated through toll-like receptors (TLRs) and produce chemokines that attract and retain additional dendritic cells (15, 16). In experimental models of vascular inflammation, activation of TLR4 was able to trigger transmural inflammation whereas activation of TLR5 induced adventitial inflammation only (17). How this relates to GCA is still uncertain. Once activated, dendritic cells are enabled to process and present antigens and express co-stimulatory molecules (CD83 and CD86) for T-cell activation (15, 16). The involvement of antigen-specific adaptive immune responses is supported by the detection of oligoclonal T-cell clones in temporal artery biopsies (18). After antigen recognition, both Th1 and Th17 differentiation pathways seem to be relevant to the pathogenesis of GCA (Figure 2.2). IFNγ is markedly and selectively expressed in GCA-involved arteries (19, 20) and its functional relevance is supported by the expression of many interferon-induced products including MHC class II antigens (14), endothelial adhesion molecules (21), inducible nitric oxide synthase (22), and chemokines (20, 23). Some of the most relevant functions of IFNγ are macrophage activation, stimulation of granuloma formation, and macrophage differentiation into giant cells (Figure 2.3). As discussed below, activated macrophages orchestrate a variety of subsequent inflammatory cascades. These are crucial to the development of full-blown transmural inflammatory infiltrates, vascular wall injury, and remodelling, which constitute the pathological substrate of the clinical symptoms and complications of GCA (3, 4, 14, 20, 22). In recent years, it has become apparent that Th17-mediated mechanisms also contribute to GCA (17, 24). CD161-positive CD4T lymphocytes, which are precursors of Th1 and Th17 functional subsets, can be identified in inflammatory infiltrates (25). Cytokines contributing to Th17 differentiation such as interleukin (IL)-1, IL-6, IL-21, and transforming growth factor beta (TGFβ) have been detected in GCA (6, 20, 24–27). IL-17A is profusely expressed in inflammatory lesions (28) (Figure 2.2). It is a highly pro-inflammatory

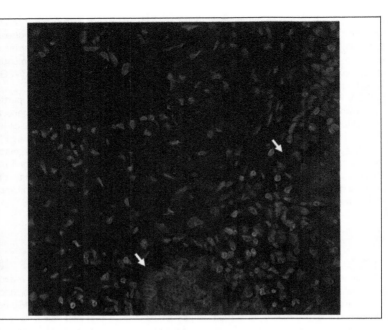

Figure 2.2 Multinucleated giant cells, the hallmark of GCA lesions (arrows). Nuclear fluorescent staining (Hoechst) examined under confocal microscopy.

cytokine with pleiotropic effects on a variety of cell types including macrophages, neutrophils, endothelial cells, and fibroblasts and actively contributes to inflammatory cascades. Both Th1 and Th17 lymphocytes are increased in peripheral blood from patients with GCA where a Th1–Th17 double-positive cell population can also be detected (25, 29). IL-17A expression rapidly and remarkably decreases upon glucocorticoid treatment suggesting that IL-17A suppression may explain the dramatic symptomatic improvement that

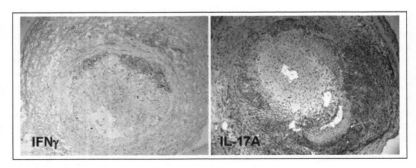

Figure 2.3 (See colour plate section). Strong expression of IFNγ and IL-17A in GCA lesions indicates the participation of both Th1- and Th17-mediated immune response pathways. Immunostaining with a mouse monoclonal antibody against human IFNγ (clone 25718.11, R&D Systems) and a goat anti-human IL-17A antibody (R&D Systems).

most patients with GCA experience with high-dose glucocorticoids (28). Patients with prominent Th17 response seem to respond better to glucocorticoids and are at a lower risk for relapses (28).

Regulatory T cells, limiting immune activation and the ensuing inflammatory response are also present in vascular lesions. In peripheral blood from patients with GCA, however, they are decreased (27, 28). In a strong inflammatory microenvironment, such as GCA inflammatory lesions, regulatory T cells may not be suppressive and may produce IL-17A (28).

2.4 Other cell types contributing to giant cell arteritis pathogenesis

The role of B cells for GCA pathogenesis has been neglected for years. However, B lymphocytes are present in vascular inflammatory lesions (14, 30, 31) and may play an even more important role in lymph nodes. Decreased concentrations of circulating B lymphocytes have been observed in patients with active GCA, which recover after treatment (30). Although GCA has primarily been considered as a T-cell-mediated disease, B lymphocytes are seminal to T-cell activation. Consistent with the potential involvement of B cells, a few reports refer to the improvement of relapsing GCA patients after B-cell depletion therapy with rituximab (33). Several autoantibodies have been detected in sera from patients with GCA including antiferritin antibodies and anti-endothelial or antivascular smooth muscle cell antibodies recognizing various antigens (i.e. vinculin and annexin V, among others) (34, 35). However, disease specificity, and the consequent diagnostic performance of these antibodies have not yet been validated. It is likely that they are generated as a consequence of inflammation and tissue injury rather than playing a primary pathogenic role. More recently, circulating autoantibodies against 14-3-3, a pleiotropic protein in nucleated cells, have been detected in patients with large-vessel vasculitis (36). The biological significance and diagnostic performance of these autoantibodies awaits wider validation.

Neutrophils are scarce in GCA transmural inflammatory infiltrates but are clearly present in small vessels surrounding the temporal artery and in early inflammatory infiltrates surrounding vasa vasorum (37, 38). Recently, changes in the phenotype of circulating neutrophils have been detected in patients with GCA. In patients treated with high-dose glucocorticoids, neutrophils have lower membrane expression of integrin CD11b, are less adhesive to endothelial cells, and are able to suppress T-cell proliferation. These abnormalities revert when glucocorticoids are tapered along with the rebound in elevated serum concentrations of IL-6, IL-8, and IL-17 which are able to induce a pro-inflammatory phenotype in neutrophils *in vitro* (39).

2.5 Amplification cascades

Following these initiating events, magnifying loops are seminal in the development and progression of transmural inflammatory infiltrates in GCA (Figure 2.4). IFNγ is a potent activator of macrophages, which are crucial in enhancing inflammatory cascades. Pro-inflammatory macrophages produce cytokines with prominent local and systemic effects and with a strong impact on disease manifestations and outcome. TNFα, IL-1β, IL-6, and IL-33 are expressed in GCA lesions and their expression correlates with the

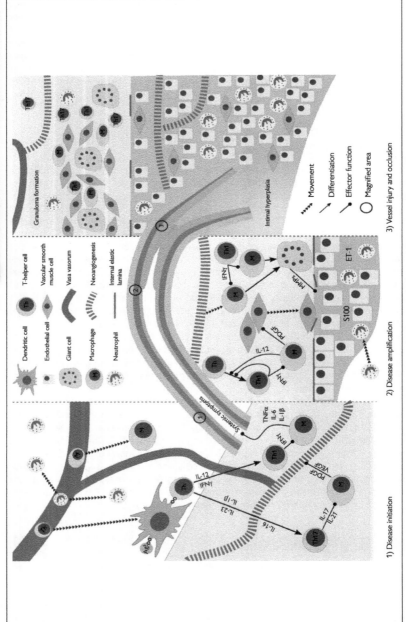

Figure 2.4 Continued

Figure 2.4 (See colour plate section). The pathophysiology of GCA disease initiation and progression. (1) Disease initiation: in response to an unknown antigen, dendritic cells within the vessel adventitia activate CD4+ helper T cells. An IL-12- and IFN-promoted Th1 response develops typified by IFNγ production, resulting in phagocyte recruitment and activation (neutrophils and macrophages). In addition, an IL-1β, IL-23-, and IL-6-promoted Th17 response develops, further enhancing phagocyte activation. Both of these responses may originate from a common CD161+ progenitor helper T-cell population. Release of pro-inflammatory cytokines into the systemic circulation, including TNFα, and IL-6 produce the systemic symptoms of GCA. Locally, vascular growth factors including PDGF and VEGF encourage neoangiogenesis within the medial layer, providing a further portal for immune cell recruitment. (2) Disease amplification: IFNγ and IL-12, produced by activated Th1 lymphocytes and macrophages, perpetuate the Th1 response. IFNγ promotes the formation of multinucleated giant cells, which continue to produce pro-inflammatory cytokines and growth factors. MMPs are produced that fragment the internal elastic lamina, while PDGF contributes to vascular smooth muscle cell activation and migration into the intimal layer. Here, vascular smooth muscle cells promote endothelial proliferation. (3) Vessel injury and occlusion: a panarteritis develops with an inflammatory infiltrate in all three layers of the vessel wall. Giant cells and granulomata form within the medial layer along the now fractured internal elastic lamina. Neoangiogenesis continues within the intimal layer, while a highly hyperplastic intima causes vessel occlusion. In larger vessels, particularly the aorta, damage to the vessel wall eventually leads to aneurysm formation. Ag, antigen; ET-1 endothelin-1; GCA, giant cell arteritis; IFNγ, interferon gamma; IL, interleukin; MMP, matrix metalloproteinase; PDGF, platelet-derived growth factor; Th, T-helper cell; TNFα tumour necrosis factor alpha; VEGF, vascular endothelial growth factor. With kind permission from Springer Science & Business Media, Drugs & Aging, Giant Cell Arteritis: Beyond Corticosteroids, Vol 32, 2015, Lauren Steel.

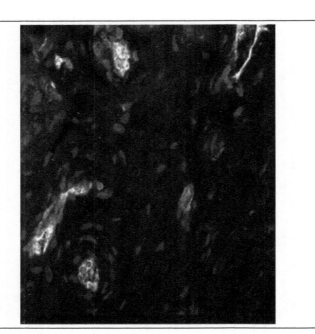

Figure 2.5 (See colour plate section). Neovascularization is a prominent finding in GCA lesions. Endothelial cell immunofluorescence staining with a mouse monoclonal antibody against CD31 (clone JC70A, Dako).

intensity of the systemic inflammatory response, which is characteristic for GCA (26, 40). Moreover, tissue expression of TNFα and circulating TNFα and IL-6 correlate with relapses and disease persistence (26). Chemokines, endothelial adhesion molecules, and colony-stimulating factors are also produced in GCA lesions and reinforce inflammatory loops by continuously recruiting and expanding the half-life of additional inflammatory cells (19, 21, 23). Angiogenic factors such as VEGF, fibroblast growth factor 2, and platelet-derived growth factors (PDGFs) promote neovascularization providing new vascular entries for infiltrating leucocytes and sustaining the active metabolic demands of the inflammatory process (3, 21, 41, 42) (Figure 2.5). In addition to fostering the progression of inflammation, angiogenesis may have a protective role by compensating for ischaemia at distal sites, and a strong angiogenic response has been associated with a lower frequency of neuro-ophthalmic ischaemic complications (43, 44).

2.6 Vascular injury

Activated macrophages produce reactive oxygen species contributing to oxidative damage and vessel wall injury (22). Matrix metalloprotease (MMP)9 and MMP2 have elastinolytic activity and are up-regulated in GCA lesions whereas their natural inhibitors tissue inhibitor of metalloproteinase (TIMP)1 and TIMP2 are down-regulated, yielding an increase in the proteolytic balance. Increased MMP9/MMP2 proteolytic activity has been demonstrated in GCA lesions and it is assumed that these factors contribute to the disruption of elastic fibres and abnormal vascular remodelling (45). Disruption of elastic fibres may favour aortic dilatation, an increasingly recognized late complication in patients with GCA (46, 47).

Currently, the treatment of GCA mainly relies on glucocorticoids, promoting a rapid relief of symptoms but failing to induce sustained remission in 60–70% of patients (48). Moreover, glucocorticoids are unable to avoid aortic dilatation in 25–30% of patients (46, 49). Understanding the pathogenic mechanisms leading to GCA may lead to the identification of better therapeutic agents. The association between increased expression of TNFα and persistent disease activity observed in various studies (26, 50) provided support to the performance of clinical trials on TNF blocking agents such as infliximab, etanercept, and adalimumab. Unfortunately, all these drugs are insufficient to abrogate inflammation and maintain remission in GCA, presumably due to redundancy in concomitantly activated inflammatory pathways (51–53). Blocking the IL-6 receptor with tocilizumab is currently being tested in a large international multicentre trial (54). IL-6 is a multifunctional cytokine involved not only in the acute phase response and systemic manifestations in GCA but also in inducing Th17 differentiation and promoting B-cell functions. IL-1β and IL-17A are additional potential targets in GCA. As mentioned earlier, both cytokines are potent pro-inflammatory molecules profusely expressed in GCA lesions. Moreover, IL-1 receptor antagonist deficiency results in large-vessel arteritis in a mouse model (55). Mice deficient in IRF-4 binding protein leading to increased expression of IL-21 and IL-17A develop large-vessel vasculitis as well (27). Proof-of-concept pilot studies testing IL-1β and IL-17 antagonism are ongoing. Interfering with CD28-mediated T-cell co-stimulation using abatacept, presumably during antigen presentation, is also currently tested in a multicentre trial (http://www.clinicaltrials.gov).

2.7 Vascular remodelling and occlusion

Growth factors produced by activated macrophages or by injured vascular smooth muscle cells drive a vascular remodelling programme leading to differentiation of smooth muscle cells into myofibroblasts, migration of these cells towards the intimal layer, and deposition of extracellular matrix proteins. This results in intimal hyperplasia and vessel occlusion. Several factors including PDGFs, TGFβ, and endothelin-1 may contribute to myofibroblast activation and production of matrix, eventually leading to vascular occlusion (24, 42, 56, 57). Blocking PDGF receptor signalling with imatinib mesylate resulted in reduced myointimal cell growth in cultured arteries (42). Increased circulating concentrations of endothelin 1 have been detected in patients with neuro-ophthalmic ischaemic complications (57). Recently, neurotrophin nerve growth factor (NGF) and brain-derived neurotrophic factor (BDNF) were identified in GCA lesions. NGF and BDNF are able to promote proliferation and migration of vascular smooth muscle cells. Consequently, the involvement of these cytokines in the generation of intimal hyperplasia has been proposed (58). Since the expression of some of these factors (i.e. TGFβ and PDGF) is not down-regulated by glucocorticoids, their specific targeting may be necessary to prevent vessel stenosis and vascular occlusion (20, 24).

2.8 Synovial inflammation in polymyalgia rheumatica

Until its anatomical substrate was characterized, PMR was clinically defined as a syndrome consisting of aches and stiffness in the upper and lower girdles (1, 11, 59). The nature of PMR symptoms was unclear for many years until imaging techniques became widely available (1, 59, 60). PMR designation reflects that muscles were the initial focus of attention as a putative target structure, but muscle biopsies never disclosed specific inflammatory findings (61). Early scintigraphy studies, and more recently ultrasonography, magnetic resonance imaging, and positron emission tomography, suggested that PMR was a disease of joints and peri-articular structures (60). It is now clear that glenohumeral synovitis, subacromial and subdeltoid bursitis, and biceps tenosynovitis underlie upper girdle pain and stiffness and that coxofemoral synovitis, iliopsoas bursitis, and, particularly, trochanteric bursitis, account for lower girdle symptoms (1, 60). Imaging has also revealed that cervical and lumbar interspinous bursitis is common and may explain neck and lumbar aches and rigidity, which are also common in PMR (62). Scattered published arthroscopic examinations have confirmed synovial inflammation which is milder than that observed in rheumatoid arthritis. Main macroscopic findings include synovial erythema, oedema, and vascular dilatation. Effusion is infrequent (63, 64).

The immunopathogenesis of synovial inflammation in PMR is less well understood than vascular immunopathology in GCA, due to the scarce availability of synovial tissue for immunopathology and molecular biology studies. Several abnormalities observed in peripheral blood mononuclear cell subsets from patients with GCA also occur in patients with PMR. An increase in circulating senescent T cells, increased numbers of Th17 lymphocytes, and decreased number of regulatory T cells have been observed in peripheral blood of both GCA and PMR patients (6, 24, 25, 29). Similarly, increased serum concentrations of IL-6 are characteristic for both conditions (44, 50, 65–67). VEGF plasma concentrations are also elevated in GCA (68) and PMR (69). More recently, by screening various potential biomarkers, elevated serum B-cell activation factor and chemokine CXCL9 have also been detected in both GCA and PMR (70).

Scarce existing immunopathology studies have revealed that synovial inflammatory infiltrates are mainly composed by memory T lymphocytes (CD45RO) and monocytes (71). Perivascular infiltrates are common, B lymphocytes and natural killer cells have not been observed so far. Infiltrating cells strongly express HLA-DR, which is lower in samples from glucocorticoid-treated patients (71). Neovessels express adhesion molecules, including P-selectin, E-selectin, intercellular adhesion molecule (ICAM)-1 and vascular cell adhesion molecule (VCAM)-1. ICAM-1 and VCAM-1 are also produced by infiltrating mononuclear cells and by synovial lining cells, Expression of adhesion molecules is weaker in samples from treated individuals (72). VEGF expression is prominent and correlates with neovascularization (69). Other authors have investigated neuropeptide expression (P substance, somatostatin, vasoactive intestinal peptide (VIP) and calcitonin gene-related peptide) and have observed VIP expression in PMR synovial tissue (73). Studies performed with PMR synovial tissue are scattered and insufficient to get convincing clues in order to elaborate a pathogenesis model. The performance of ultrasound-guided biopsies in patients with PMR may allow, through multicentre collaboration, the performance of immunopathology and biomarker studies leading to a significant advance in understanding PMR pathogenesis.

2.9 **Concluding remarks**

PMR and GCA are closely related conditions, probably sharing common immunopathogenic mechanisms and predisposing factors. Activated immune and inflammatory pathways may target vascular or synovial tissue independently, concomitantly, or sequentially. Glucocorticoids are the cornerstone of treatment in both diseases, achieving a remarkable symptomatic relief. However, glucocorticoids are unable to induce sustained remission in a substantial proportion of individuals and frequently result in severe or disturbing side effects. A better understanding of immunopathogenic mechanisms leading to the development and progression of synovial and vascular inflammation, as well as to vascular remodelling, is crucial to the identification of finely targeted, more efficient, and safer therapies.

Acknowledgement

Supported by Ministerio de Economía y Competitividad (SAF 2014/57708-R).

References

1. Salvarani C, Pipitone N, Versari A, et al. Clinical features of polymyalgia rheumatica and giant cell arteritis. Nat Rev Rheumatol 2012; 8:509–21.

2. Hernández-Rodríguez J, Font C, García-Martínez A, et al. Development of ischemic complications in patients with giant cell arteritis presenting with apparently isolated polymyalgia rheumatica: study of a series of 100 patients. Medicine (Baltimore) 2007; 86:233–41.

3. Cid MC, Font C, Coll-Vinent B, et al. Large vessel vasculitides. Curr Opin Rheumatol 1998; 10:18–28.

4. Weyand CM, Goronzy JJ. Immune mechanisms in medium and large-vessel vasculitis. Nat Rev Rheumatol 2013; 9:731–40.

5. González-Gay MA, Martinez-Dubois C, Agudo M, et al. Giant cell arteritis: epidemiology, diagnosis, and management. Curr Rheumatol Rep 2010; 12:436–42.

6. Dejaco C, Duftner C, Al-Massad J, et al. NKG2D stimulated T-cell autoreactivity in giant cell arteritis and polymyalgia rheumatica. Ann Rheum Dis 2013; 72:1852–9.

7. Liozon E, Ouattara B, Rhaiem K, et al. Familial aggregation in giant cell arteritis and polymyalgia rheumatica: a comprehensive literature review including 4 new families. Clin Exp Rheumatol 2009; 27(1 Suppl 52):S89–94.

8. Carmona FD, González-Gay MA, Martín J. Genetic component of giant cell arteritis. Rheumatology (Oxford) 2014; 53:6–18.

9. Serrano A, Márquez A, Mackie SL, et al; UK GCA Consortium Spanish GCA Consortium. Identification of the PTPN22 functional variant R620W as susceptibility genetic factor for giant cell arteritis. Ann Rheum Dis 2013; 72:1882–6.

10. Enjuanes A, Benavente Y, Hernández-Rodríguez J, et al. Association of NOS2 and potential effect of VEGF, IL6, CCL2 and IL1RN polymorphisms and haplotypes on susceptibility to GCA – a simultaneous study of 130 potentially functional SNPs in 14 candidate genes. Rheumatology (Oxford) 2012; 51:841–51.

11. Dasgupta B, Cimmino MA, Maradit-Kremers H, et al. 2012 provisional classification criteria for polymyalgia rheumatica: a European League Against Rheumatism/American College of Rheumatology collaborative initiative. Ann Rheum Dis 2012; 71:484–92.

12. Carmona FD, Mackie SL, Martín JE, et al. A large-scale genetic analysis reveals a strong contribution of the HLA class II region to giant cell arteritis susceptibility. Am J Hum Genet 2015; 96:565–80.

13. Bhatt AS, Manzo VE, Pedamallu CS, et al. In search of a candidate pathogen for giant cell arteritis: sequencing-based characterization of the giant cell arteritis microbiome. Arthritis Rheumatol 2014; 66:1939–44.

14. Cid MC, Campo E, Ercilla G, et al. Immunohistochemical analysis of lymphoid and macrophage cell subsets and their immunologic activation markers in temporal arteritis. Influence of corticosteroid treatment. Arthritis Rheum 1989; 32:884–93.

15. Krupa WM, Dewan M, Jeon MS, et al. Trapping of misdirected dendritic cells in the granu-lomatous lesions of giant cell arteritis. Am J Pathol 2002; 161:1815–23.

16. Ma-Krupa W, Jeon MS, Spoerl S, et al. Activation of arterial wall dendritic cells and break-down of self-tolerance in giant cell arteritis. J Exp Med 2004; 199:173–83.

17. Deng J, Ma-Krupa W, Gewirtz AT, et al. Toll-like receptors 4 and 5 induce distinct types of vasculitis. Circ Res 2009; 104:488–95.

18. Weyand CM, Schönberger J, Oppitz U, et al. Distinct vascular lesions in giant cell arteritis share identical T cell clonotypes. J Exp Med 1994; 179(3):951–60.

19. Weyand CM, Hicok KC, Hunder GG, et al. Tissue cytokine patterns in patients with polymy-algia rheumatica and giant cell arteritis. Ann Intern Med 1994; 121:484–91.

20. Corbera-Bellalta M, García-Martínez A, Lozano E, et al. Changes in biomarkers after thera-peutic intervention in temporal arteries cultured in Matrigel: a new model for preclinical stud-ies in giant-cell arteritis. Ann Rheum Dis 2014; 73:616–23.

21. Cid MC, Cebrián M, Font C, et al. Cell adhesion molecules in the development of inflamma-tory infiltrates in giant cell arteritis: inflammation-induced angiogenesis as the preferential site of leukocyte-endothelial cell interactions. Arthritis Rheum 2000; 43:184–94.

22. Weyand CM, Wagner AD, Björnsson J, et al. Correlation of the topographical arrangement and the functional pattern of tissue-infiltrating macrophages in giant cell arteritis. J Clin Invest 1996; 98:1642–9.

23. Cid MC, Hoffman MP, Hernández-Rodríguez J, et al. Association between increased CCL2 (MCP-1) expression in lesions and persistence of disease activity in giant-cell arteritis. Rheumatology (Oxford) 2006; 45:1356–63.

24. Espígol-Frigolé G, Corbera-Bellalta M, Planas-Rigol E, et al. Increased IL-17A expression in temporal artery lesions is a predictor of sustained response to glucocorticoid treatment in patients with giant-cell arteritis. Ann Rheum Dis 2013; 72:1481–7.

25. Visvanathan S, Rahman MU, Hoffman GS, et al. Tissue and serum markers of inflammation during the follow-up of patients with giant-cell arteritis--a prospective longitudinal study. Rheumatology (Oxford) 2011; 50:2061–70.

26. Samson M, Audia S, Fraszczak J, et al. Th1 and Th17 lymphocytes expressing CD161 are implicated in giant cell arteritis and polymyalgia rheumatica pathogenesis. Arthritis Rheum 2012; 64:3788–98.

27. Hernández-Rodríguez J, Segarra M, Vilardell C, et al. Tissue production of pro-inflammatory cytokines (IL-1beta, TNF alpha and IL-6) correlates with the intensity of the systemic inflam-matory response and with corticosteroid requirements in giant-cell arteritis. Rheumatology (Oxford) 2004; 43:294–301.

28. Terrier B, Geri G, Chaara W, et al. Interleukin-21 modulates Th1 and Th17 responses in giant cell arteritis. Arthritis Rheum 2012; 64:2001–11.

29. Deng J, Younge BR, Olshen RA, et al. Th17 and Th1 T-cell responses in giant cell arteritis. Circulation 2010; 121(7):906–15.

30. van der Geest KS, Abdulahad WH, Chalan P, et al. Disturbed B cell homeostasis in newly diag-nosed giant cell arteritis and polymyalgia rheumatica. Arthritis Rheumatol 2014; 66:1927–38.

31. Alba MA, Prieto-González S, Hernández-Rodríguez J, et al. B lymphocytes may play a signifi-cant role in large-vessel vasculitis. Int J Clin Rheumatol 2012; 7:475–7.

32. Bhatia A, Ell PJ, Edwards JC. Anti-CD20 monoclonal antibody (rituximab) as an adjunct in the treatment of giant cell arteritis. Ann Rheum Dis 2005; 64:1099–100.

33. Alba MA, Espígol-Frigolé G, Butjosa M, et al. Treatment of large-vessel vasculitis. Curr Immunol Rev 2011; 7:435–42.

34. Baerlecken NT, Linnemann A, Gross WL, et al. Association of ferritin autoantibodies with giant cell arteritis/polymyalgia rheumatica. Ann Rheum Dis 2012; 71:943–7.

35. Régent A, Dib H, Ly KH, et al. Identification of target antigens of anti-endothelial cell and anti-vascular smooth muscle cell antibodies in patients with giant cell arteritis: a proteomic approach. Arthritis Res Ther 2011; 13:R107.

36. Chakravarti R, Gupta K, Swain M, et al. 14-3-3 in thoracic aortic aneurysms: Identification of a novel auto-antigen in large vessel vasculitis. Arthritis Rheumatol 2015; 67(7):1913–21.

37. Esteban MJ, Font C, Hernández-Rodríguez J, et al. Small-vessel vasculitis surrounding a spared temporal artery: clinical and pathological findings in a series of twenty-eight patients. Arthritis Rheum 2001; 44:1387–95.

38. Foell D, Hernández-Rodríguez J, Sánchez M, et al. Early recruitment of phagocytes contributes to the vascular inflammation of giant cell arteritis. J Pathol 2004; 204:311–16.

39. Nadkarni S, Dalli J, Hollywood J, et al. Investigational analysis reveals a potential role for neutrophils in giant-cell arteritis disease progression. Circ Res 2014; 114:242–8.

40. Ciccia F, Alessandro R, Rizzo A, et al. IL-33 is overexpressed in the inflamed arteries of patients with giant cell arteritis. Ann Rheum Dis 2013; 72:258–64.

41. Kaiser M, Younge B, Björnsson J, et al. Formation of new vasa vasorum in vasculitis. Production of angiogenic cytokines by multinucleated giant cells. Am J Pathol 1999; 155:765–74.

42. Lozano E, Segarra M, García-Martínez A, et al. Imatinib mesylate inhibits in vitro and ex vivo biological responses related to vascular occlusion in giant cell arteritis. Ann Rheum Dis 2008; 67:1581–8.

43. Cid MC, Hernández-Rodríguez J, Esteban MJ, et al. Tissue and serum angiogenic activity is associated with low prevalence of ischemic complications in patients with giant-cell arteritis. Circulation 2002; 106:1664–71.

44. Hernández-Rodríguez J, Segarra M, Vilardell C, et al. Elevated production of interleukin-6 is associated with a lower incidence of disease-related ischemic events in patients with giant-cell arteritis: angiogenic activity of interleukin-6 as a potential protective mechanism. Circulation 2003; 107(19):2428–34.

45. Segarra M, García-Martínez A, Sánchez M, et al. Gelatinase expression and proteolytic activity in giant-cell arteritis. Ann Rheum Dis 2007; 66:1429–35.

46. Kermani TA, Warrington KJ, Crowson CS, et al. Large-vessel involvement in giant cell arteritis: a population-based cohort study of the incidence-trends and prognosis. Ann Rheum Dis 2013; 72:1989–94.

47. García-Martínez A, Hernández-Rodríguez J, Arguis P, et al. Development of aortic aneurysm/ dilatation during the followup of patients with giant cell arteritis: a cross-sectional screening of fifty-four prospectively followed patients. Arthritis Rheum 2008; 59:422–30.

48. Alba MA, García-Martínez A, Prieto-González S, et al. Relapses in patients with giant cell arteritis: prevalence, characteristics, and associated clinical findings in a longitudinally followed cohort of 106 patients. Medicine (Baltimore) 2014; 93:194–201.

49. García-Martínez A, Arguis P, Prieto-González S, et al. Prospective long term follow-up of a cohort of patients with giant cell arteritis screened for aortic structural damage (aneurysm or dilatation). Ann Rheum Dis 2014; 73:1826–32.

50. García-Martínez A, Hernández-Rodríguez J, Espígol-Frigolé G, et al. Clinical relevance of persistently elevated circulating cytokines (tumor necrosis factor alpha and interleukin-6) in the long-term followup of patients with giant cell arteritis. Arthritis Care Res (Hoboken) 2010; 62:835–41.

51. Hoffman GS, Cid MC, Rendt-Zagar KE, et al; Infliximab-GCA Study Group. Infliximab for maintenance of glucocorticosteroid-induced remission of giant cell arteritis: a randomized trial. Ann Intern Med 2007; 146:621–30.

52. Martínez-Taboada VM, Rodríguez-Valverde V, Carreño L, et al. A double-blind placebo controlled trial of etanercept in patients with giant cell arteritis and corticosteroid side effects. Ann Rheum Dis 2008; 67:625–30.

53. Seror R, Baron G, Hachulla E, et al. Adalimumab for steroid sparing in patients with giant-cell arteritis: results of a multicentre randomised controlled trial. Ann Rheum Dis 2014; 73:2074–81.

54. Unizony SH, Dasgupta B, Fisheleva E, et al. Design of the tocilizumab in giant cell arteritis trial. Int J Rheumatol 2013; 2103:912562.

55. Nicklin MJ, Hughes DE, Barton JL, et al. Arterial inflammation in mice lacking the interleukin 1 receptor antagonist gene. J Exp Med 2000; 191:303–12.

56. Kaiser M, Weyand CM, Björnsson J, et al. Platelet-derived growth factor, intimal hyperplasia, and ischemic complications in giant cell arteritis. Arthritis Rheum 1998; 41:623–33.

57. Lozano E, Segarra M, Corbera-Bellalta M, et al. Increased expression of the endothelin system in arterial lesions from patients with giant-cell arteritis: association between elevated plasma endothelin levels and the development of ischaemic events. Ann Rheum Dis 2010; 69:434–42.

58. Ly K, Régent A, Molina E, et al. Neurotrophins are expressed in giant-cell arteritis lesions and may contribute to vascular remodeling. Arthritis Res Ther 2014; 16:487.

59. Kermani TA, Warrington KJ. Polymyalgia rheumatica. Lancet 2013; 381:63–72.

60. Camellino D, Cimmino MA. Imaging of polymyalgia rheumatica: indications on its pathogenesis, diagnosis and prognosis. Rheumatology (Oxford) 2012; 51:77–86.

61. Bruk MI. Articular and vascular manifestations of polymyalgia rheumatica. Ann Rheum Dis 1967; 26:103–16.

62. Salvarani C, Barozzi L, Cantini F, et al. Cervical interspinous bursitis in active polymyalgia rheumatica. Ann Rheum Dis 2008; 67:758–61.

63. Chou CT, Schumacher HR Jr. Clinical and pathologic studies of synovitis in polymyalgia rheumatica. Arthritis Rheum 1984; 27:1107–17.

64. Douglas WA, Martin BA, Morris JH. Polymyalgia rheumatica: an arthroscopic study of the shoulder joint. Ann Rheum Dis 1983; 42:311–16.

65. Dasgupta B, Panayi GS. Interleukin-6 in serum of patients with polymyalgia rheumatica and giant cell arteritis. Br J Rheumatol 1990; 29:456–8.

66. Hernández-Rodríguez J, García-Martínez A, Casademont J, et al. A strong initial systemic inflammatory response is associated with higher corticosteroid requirements and longer duration of therapy in patients with giant-cell arteritis. Arthritis Rheum 2002; 47:29–35.

67. Martinez-Taboada VM, Alvarez L, Ruiz Soto M, et al. Giant cell arteritis and polymyalgia rheumatica: role of cytokines in the pathogenesis and implications for treatment. Cytokine 2008; 44:207–20.

68. Baldini M, Maugeri N, Ramirez GA, et al. Selective up-regulation of the soluble pattern-recognition receptor pentraxin 3 and of vascular endothelial growth factor in giant cell arteritis: relevance for recent optic nerve ischemia. Arthritis Rheum 2012; 64:854–65.

69. Meliconi R, Pulsatelli L, Dolzani P, et al. Vascular endothelial growth factor production in polymyalgia rheumatica. Arthritis Rheum 2000; 43:2472–80.

70. van der Geest KS, Abdulahad WH, Rutgers A, et al. Serum markers associated with disease activity in giant cell arteritis and polymyalgia rheumatica. Rheumatology (Oxford). 2015; 54(8):1397–402.

71. Meliconi R, Pulsatelli L, Uguccioni M, et al. Leukocyte infiltration in synovial tissue from the shoulder of patients with polymyalgia rheumatica. Quantitative analysis and influence of corticosteroid treatment. Arthritis Rheum 1996; 39:1199–207.

72. Meliconi R, Pulsatelli L, Melchiorri C, et al. Synovial expression of cell adhesion molecules in polymyalgia rheumatica. Clin Exp Immunol 1997; 107:494–500.

73. Pulsatelli L, Dolzani P, Silvestri T, et al. Synovial expression of vasoactive intestinal peptide in polymyalgia rheumatica. Clin Exp Rheumatol 2006; 24:562–6.

Chapter 3

Clinical presentation and classification criteria for polymyalgia rheumatica

Wiliam Docken, Eric L. Matteson, and Bhaskar Dasgupta

Key points

- Polymyalgia rheumatica (PMR) affects only older adults, most commonly in the seventh decade, and is significantly more prevalent in white than non-white populations.

- The clinical presentation of PMR is dominated by proximal stiffness of new onset, worst about the arms, hips, and neck, which is particularly prominent on awakening.

- Provisional European League Against Rheumatism/American College of Rheumatology classification criteria for PMR have the highest sensitivity and specificity of published classification criteria. Inclusion of ultrasound abnormalities seen in synovial structures of the proximal joints and bursae increases both sensitivity and specificity to over 90%.

3.1 Introduction

The essential outlines of the clinical presentation of PMR can be sketched with a few strokes: an older adult, proximally distributed aching, an abrupt onset, and prominent morning stiffness. In this chapter, we will fill in this clinical portrait of PMR, and present proposed criteria for its classification.

3.2 Background

The clinical portrait of PMR begins with demographics, of which two features are key, namely age and ethnicity. PMR, like its companion giant cell arteritis (GCA), is the quintessential systemic rheumatic disease of older adults. The mean age at the time of diagnosis is 74 years. PMR occurs rarely, if at all, in patients under the age of 50 years. It becomes more common with increasing age. The prevalence peaks in the seventh decade, and new cases can occur in patients in their 90s (1).

The second key feature is ethnicity: though all racial and ethnic groups can be affected, the disease is far more common in white than in non-white people. The incidence is highest in individuals of Scandinavian descent, and is decidedly unusual in patients of African American, Latin, and Asian heritage (2–4).

Women are affected two to three times more frequently than men, and have a higher lifetime risk for developing PMR (2.4%) than men (1.7%) (5).

3.3 Onset

The onset of symptoms in PMR is often abrupt. Patients may cite a given week or weekend when their symptoms commenced. An occasional patient reports symptoms that seem to have appeared overnight. Whatever the celerity of onset, the important point is that the onset of PMR involves a discrete change in musculoskeletal symptoms and, commonly, a rapid decline in function. A history of long-standing aching and stiffness would be exceptional. The abruptness of onset often prompts the patient to propose a provocative event—unusual physical activity, a new medication, or a recent illness—but no one historical feature is consistently observed.

3.4 **Constitutional symptoms**

Musculoskeletal symptoms can be accompanied by some degree of low-grade fatigue, malaise, and depression. Significant constitutional symptoms in uncomplicated PMR, however, are uncommon. Explicit, persisting fever and major weight loss are unusual, and should raise concerns for associated GCA, infection, or malignancy.

3.5 **Pattern of symptoms**

The full picture of PMR classically manifests with symptoms about the upper arms, posterior neck, and pelvic girdle. Symptoms affecting the arms and legs are bilateral and symmetric; unilateral shoulder pain of recent onset in an older adult does not suggest the presence of PMR. Involvement of the upper arms is especially common in PMR, and frequently dominates the clinical presentation, especially early in the clinical course. Very occasionally, proximal lower extremity symptoms—again, bilateral and symmetric—predominate, with but minor background symptoms about the upper arms and posterior neck. Pelvic girdle symptoms affect the hips anteriorly, laterally, and posteriorly, and are often described as radiating to the posterior thighs.

In addition to the proximally distributed symptomatology, distal musculoskeletal symptoms occur in PMR, and, if sought, can be found in up to one-half of patients (6). Such symptoms are most common at the wrists and metacarpophalangeal joints, and, less frequently, at the knees. The feet are virtually never involved. Distal findings also include symptoms referable to carpal tunnel syndromes, secondary to wrist involvement, which may occur in up to 15% of patients (6). Distal involvement at the wrists and hands occasionally is explosive and exuberant (see section 3.8).

3.6 **The gel phenomenon**

Morning stiffness is a cardinal clinical symptom of most systemic rheumatic diseases. The gel phenomenon—stiffness with inactivity—is invariable in PMR, and can be notable for its severity. In untreated PMR, morning stiffness can last until the afternoon, and then frequently recrudesces with immobility, such as riding in a car or after prolonged sitting, or at night. Complaints of nocturnal pain and disrupted sleep are common.

3.7 Functional limitations

Proximal symptoms and a prominent gel phenomenon can affect activities of daily living. Stiffness of the shoulders can cause difficulty hooking a bra in the back, or donning a shirt or coat; stiffness about the hips can similarly affect reaching for socks and shoes. Transfers out of bed in the morning, or from a toilet or deep couch, can be challenging.

These functional limitations are not unique to PMR, and can arise from other musculoskeletal conditions with proximal involvement, such as rotator cuff pathology at the shoulders or osteoarthritis at the hips, but their magnitude can be striking in PMR, and are mimicked in their suddenness of onset and severity by few other conditions. The symptoms may be so severe that, for instance, assistance may be required for the simple activity of putting on a bathrobe. Continued pursuit of fitness activities can be problematic. The functional limitations, in concert with the intensity of aching and stiffness, often confers an urgency to a patient's appeal for consultation that is recognizable to physicians familiar with PMR.

3.8 Directed physical examination

The proper examination of the patient with PMR can be hampered by its very name, poly*myalgia*, which implies a disease of muscles. It is, however, principally articular and periarticular structures—joints, bursae, tendons, and entheses—that are affected in PMR, rather than the muscles (see Chapter 2). Involvement of these structures is responsible for the patterns of pain referral to the upper arms and thighs in PMR. Stiffness about the spine, especially the cervical and lumbar spine, can be related to interspinous bursitis and ligament enthesitis (7, 8). Tenderness of the muscles to palpation is a sign of no particular specificity, and in the patient with PMR, muscle strength is normal, though the performance of an adequate motor examination in a patient with prominent aching and stiffness can be difficult owing to involvement of the joints and periarticular structures.

The crucial part of the physical examination in suspected PMR is therefore the joint examination. Range of motion about the shoulders, cervical spine, and hips can be limited. Restricted motion about the shoulders is common; a classic finding in PMR is an inability to abduct actively the shoulders above 90°. Distal findings, when present, are most frequent at the wrists and metacarpophalangeal joints, and are manifested by dorsal swelling, usually of a modest degree, and limited flexion and extension. Minor knee effusions can occur, but the ankles and metatarsophalangeal joints are spared.

An unusual expression of distal involvement is the puffy oedematous hand syndrome, christened the RS3PE syndrome (Figure 3.1), or *remitting seronegative symmetrical synovitis with peripheral oedema* (Figure 3.2) (9). In this syndrome, distal symptoms and signs appear suddenly. Pain and functional limitations can be marked, and swelling, which can be pitting, extends from the wrists over the dorsa of the hands to fingers, productive of a 'boxing glove' appearance. Proximal symptomatology is often less prominent. The diffuse swelling corresponds in large part to severe tenosynovitis of forearm and hand

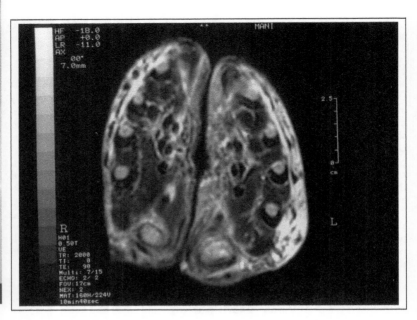

Figure 3.1 Magnetic resonance image from a patient with PMR and RS3PE syndrome. The axial T2-weighted image is taken at the midpoint of the palm. Subcutaneous oedema is present in the soft tissues of the dorsum of the hand and there is fluid representing synovitis in the extensor synovial sheaths.

extensor tendons (10). When these symptoms and signs subside briskly and completely with low-dose glucocorticoid therapy, it is reasonable to interpret the puffy oedematous hand syndrome as belonging to the clinical spectrum of PMR.

Notwithstanding a suspected clinical diagnosis of PMR, the occurrence of distal findings, particularly at the metacarpophalangeal and proximal interphalangeal joints, warrants concern for rheumatoid disease (see Chapter 9).

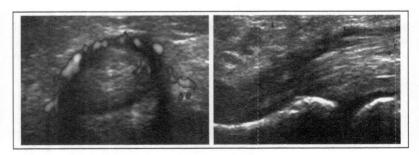

Figure 3.2 (See colour plate section). Ultrasound of hands in PMR and RS3PE. A 77-year-old man presented with polymyalgia, swollen hands, and pitting oedema—ultrasound showed power Doppler signals associated with flexor tenosynovitis.

3.9 Evaluation for giant cell arteritis

GCA and PMR may occur separately and have overlapping clinical features. Subclinical large-vessel inflammation may occur in PMR, a condition described as polymyalgia arteritica in older literature (11). If the clinical presentation suggests PMR, assessment for stigmata of GCA is mandatory. The history should include focused questions with regard to new-onset headache, new facial or dental pain, recent visual symptoms, especially transient monocular visual impairment, jaw pain, and symptoms of limb claudication. Physical examination should include measurements of blood pressures in both arms, palpation of peripheral arteries, including the superficial temporal arteries, and cardiac examination and auscultation for bruits. The general physical examination is also important for findings that are *not* part of the clinical presentation of PMR, such as skin rash, lymphadenopathy, pulmonary rales, organomegaly, or focal neuropathy (other than carpal tunnel syndrome), which would draw attention to the prospect of alternative diagnoses.

3.10 Provisional classification criteria

Several sets of criteria have been suggested for the classification and diagnosis of PMR, based primarily on the chief symptoms of PMR, bilateral pain, and stiffness of the hips and shoulders, along with elevated inflammatory markers (erythrocyte sedimentation rate and C-reactive protein) (12–14). These features have been captured in the provisional classification criteria for polymyalgia rheumatica as proposed by the European League Against Rheumatism/American College of Rheumatology (EULAR/ACR) (Table 3.1) (13).

Table 3.1 Provisional EULAR/ACR classification criteria for polymyalgia rheumatica scoring algorithm. Required criteria: age 50 years or greater, bilateral shoulder aching, and abnormal C-reactive protein and/or erythrocyte sedimentation rate

Criteria	Points without ultrasound (0–6)	Points with ultrasound* (0 = 8)
Morning stiffness duration > 45 minutes	2	2
Hip pain or limited range of movement	1	1
Absence of RF or ACPA	2	2
Absence of other joint involvement	1	1
At least 1 shoulder with subdeltoid bursitis and/or biceps tenosynovitis and/or glenohumeral synovitis (either posterior or axillary) and at least 1 hip with synovitis and/or trochanteric bursitis	n/a	1
Both shoulders with subdeltoid bursitis, biceps tenosynovitis, or glenohumeral synovitis	n/a	1

In the algorithm a score of 4 or more is categorized as polymyalgia rheumatica without ultrasound and a score of 5 or more is categorized as polymyalgia rheumatica with ultrasonographic identification of inflammatory changes typical of polymyalgia rheumatica in the shoulders and hips.

ACPA, anti-citrullinated protein antibody; n/a = not applicable; RF, rheumatoid factor.

*Optional ultrasound criteria.

Reproduced from Dasgupta B, Cimmino MA, Maradit-Kremers H, Schmidt WA, Schirmer M, Salvarani C, et al. 2012 provisional classification criteria for polymyalgia rheumatica: a European League Against Rheumatism/American College of Rheumatology collaborative initiative. 2012, Wiley.

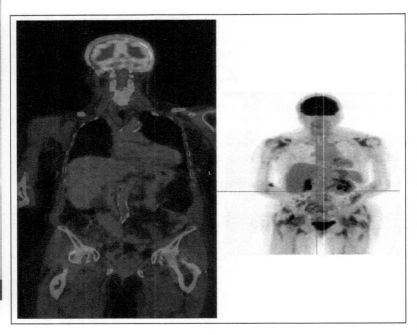

Figure 3.3 (See colour plate section). Fluorodeoxyglucose-positron emission tomography (FDG-PET) scan showing bursitis and enthesitis in PMR. A 69-year-old with severe PMR, constitutional symptoms, and high inflammatory markers underwent a FDG-PET scan to exclude alternative diagnoses. FDG-PET showed typical changes of bursitis, capsulitis, and enthesitis in multiple areas of the shoulders, hips, trochanteric, and ischial bursae.

Reproduced from Williams M, Jain S, Patil P, and Dasgupta B, Contribution of imaging in polymyalgia rheumatic, Joint Bone Spine, 2013: 80; 228–9 with permission from Elsevier.

The performance of the classification criteria are improved with inclusion of the ultrasonographic findings typical of PMR, which include glenohumeral synovitis, subdeltoid and biceps tenosynovitis, hip joint synovitis, and trochanteric bursitis (Figure 3.3). These abnormalities can be found even in the unusual cases where the acute phase reactants are normal at presentation (15). In a patient aged 50 years or over with new-onset bilateral shoulder aching, and an abnormal C-reactive protein and/or erythrocyte sedimentation rate, the ultrasonographic findings are strongly supportive of a diagnosis of PMR. However, they are also seen in rheumatoid arthritis, and thus alone cannot distinguish PMR from rheumatoid disease. The presence of rheumatoid factor or anticyclic citrullinated peptide antibodies argues against a diagnosis of PMR and prompts consideration of rheumatoid arthritis.

While intended to classify patients with PMR for research purposes, these classification criteria have been evaluated against other classification and diagnostic criteria for PMR. The EULAR/ACR criteria have highest sensitivity (93%) and comparable specificity (92%) for diagnosis of PMR (16). Addition of ultrasonographic data as outlined in Table 3.1 increases the specificity of the diagnosis to 91% (16).

References

1. Doran MF, Crowson CS, O'Fallon WM, et al. Trends in the incidence of polymyalgia rheumatica over a 30 year period in Olmsted County, Minnesota, USA. *J Rheumatol* 2001; 29:1694–7.

2. Gonzalez-Gay MA, Vazquez-Rodriguez TR, Lopez-Diaz MJ, et al. Epidemiology of giant cell arteritis and polymyalgia rheumatica. *Arthritis Rheum* 2009; 61:1454–61.

3. Boesen P, Sorensen SF. Giant cell arteritis, temporal arteritis, and polymyalgia rheumatica in a Danish county: a prospective investigation. *Arthritis Rheum* 1987; 30:294–9.

4. Salvarani C, Macchioni P, Zizzi F, et al. Epidemiologic and immunogenetic aspects of polymyalgia rheumatica and giant cell arteritis in northern Italy. *Arthritis Rheum* 1991; 34:351–6.

5. Crowson CS, Matteson EL, Myasoedova E, et al. The lifetime risk of adult-onset rheumatoid arthritis and other inflammatory autoimmune rheumatic diseases. *Arthritis Rheum* 2011; 63:633–9.

6. Salvarani C, Cantini F, Macchioni P, et al. Distal musculoskeletal manifestations in polymyalgia rheumatica: a prospective followup study. *Arthritis Rheum* 1998; 41:1221–6.

7. Salvarani C, Barozzi L, Cantini F, et al. Cervical interspinous bursitis in active polymyalgia rheumatica. *Ann Rheum Dis* 2008; 67:758–61.

8. Salvarani C, Barozzi L, Boiardi L, et al. Lumbar interspinous bursitis in active polymyalgia rheumatica. *Clin Exp Rheumatol* 2013; 31:526–31.

9. McCarty DJ, O'Duffy JD, Pearson L, et al. Remitting seronegative symmetrical synovitis with pitting edema. RS3PE syndrome. *JAMA* 1985; 254:2763–7.

10. Cantini F, Salvarani C, Olivieri I, et al. Remitting seronegative symmetrical synovitis with pitting oedema (RS3PE) syndrome: a prospective follow up and magnetic resonance imaging study. *Ann Rheum Dis* 1999; 58:230–6.

11. Hamrin B. Polymyalgia arteritica. *Acta Med Scand Suppl* 1972; 533:1–133.

12. Salvarani C, Pipitone N, Versari A, et al. Clinical features of polymyalgia rheumatica and giant cell arteritis. *Nat Rev Rheumatol* 2012; 8:509–21

13. Dasgupta B, Cimmino MA, Maradit-Kremers H, et al. 2012 provisional classification criteria for polymyalgia rheumatica: a European League Against Rheumatism/American College of Rheumatology collaborative initiative. *Ann Rheum Dis* 2012; 71:484–92.

14. Bird HA, Esselinckx W, Dixon AS, et al. An evaluation of criteria for polymyalgia rheumatica. *Ann Rheum Dis* 1979; 38:434–9.

15. Cantini F, Salvarani C, Olivieri I, et al. Inflamed shoulder structures in polymyalgia rheumatica with normal erythrocyte sedimentation rate. *Arthritis Rheum* 2001; 44:1155–9.

16. Macchioni P, Boiardi L, Catanoso M, et al. Performance of the new 2012 EULAR/ACR classification criteria for polymyalgia rheumatica: comparison with the previous criteria in a single-centre study. *Ann Rheum Dis* 2014; 73:1190–3.

Chapter 4

Clinical manifestations of giant cell arteritis

Carlo Salvarani and Nicolò Pipitone

Key points

- Giant cell arteritis (GCA) can present with a variety of symptoms and signs.
- Headache, jaw claudication, and visual symptoms should alert to a diagnosis of GCA.
- Patients with GCA may present predominantly or exclusively with constitutional manifestations and/or polymyalgia (polymyalgia arteritica).
- GCA-related ischaemic complications including visual loss can be prevented by prompt glucocorticoid therapy.

4.1 Introduction

GCA can present with a wide gamut of clinical features (Box 4.1), while additional features can develop during the course of the disease (Box 4.2). Most patients have symptoms and signs (Table 4.1) directly related to the involvement of the arteries; some patients also display constitutional manifestations that reflect the generalized inflammatory status, and some have both arteritic and constitutional manifestations (1). GCA is more common in individuals of Northern European ancestry, but its clinical manifestations are broadly similar in patients from Northern and Southern Europe (2) and from Japan (3). However, Japanese patients with GCA tend to develop polymyalgia rheumatica (PMR), jaw claudication, and visual loss less often than their Western counterparts (3).

4.2 Cranial symptoms

The most frequent initial symptom of GCA is new onset of headache (or worsening of a pre-existing headache), which affects approximately two-thirds of patients (4). The headache is usually localized to the temporal or sometimes to the occipital area, but may also be diffuse (5). It is often boring or lancinating in nature (1) and responds poorly to conventional anodynes (5). GCA-related headache is usually due to the involvement of extracranial arteries, and temporal artery abnormalities on clinical examination are more frequent in patients with cranial symptoms (6). However,

Box 4.1 Main initial clinical manifestations of GCA

- Headache (32%)
- PMR (25%)
- Fever (15%)
- Fatigue or malaise (5%)
- Visual symptoms (excluding visual loss) (7%)
- Visual loss (1%)
- Weight loss (2%)
- Temporal artery tenderness (60–70%).

in some patients headache may be quite marked even when the temporal arteries appear clinically normal (1). Half of patients with GCA also complain of dysesthesia of the scalp that is worsened by combing or brushing the hair, mostly associated with headache (4, 5).

4.3 Jaw claudication and ischaemic symptoms

Jaw claudication and ischaemic symptoms (pain on chewing) due to ischaemia of the masticatory muscles occur in about 50% of patients (4, 5). Jaw claudication is highly suggestive, but not pathognomonic of GCA, since it can rarely be a manifestation of other vasculitides or of amyloidosis. Occasionally, claudication may affect the muscles of the tongue or those involved in swallowing. When ischaemic changes are particularly severe, necrosis of the scalp, tongue, or lips may develop (5, 7). Necrotic lesions are very rare, and are often associated with ischaemic changes at other sites (such as visual loss) (7). Like most GCA-related ischaemic complications, necrosis develops mostly before the onset of glucocorticoid therapy; however, unlike visual loss, tissue necrosis resolves or improves in about three-quarters of patients once glucocorticoids are commenced (7).

4.4 Visual symptoms

One of the most dreaded, and frequent, ischaemic complications of GCA is partial or complete loss of vision in one or both eyes, which occurs in approximately 15–20%

Box 4.2 Main clinical manifestation throughout the course of GCA

- Headache (83%)
- PMR (39%)
- Fever (42%)
- Fatigue or malaise (40%)
- Visual symptoms (excluding visual loss) (68%)
- Visual loss (14%)
- Weight loss (50%)
- Temporal artery tenderness (66%).

Source data from: Calamia KT, Hunder GG. Clinical manifestations of giant cell (temporal) arteritis. *Clin Rheum Dis* 1980; 6:389–403.

Table 4.1 Common symptoms and signs of GCA

Symptoms	Signs	Differential diagnoses
• Abrupt onset headache: – usually unilateral and temporal – occasionally diffuse or bilateral. • Scalp pain: – diffuse or localised – may lead to difficulty in combing hair • Jaw and tongue claudication • Visual symptoms: – amaurosis fugax, blurring and diplopia • Constitutional symptoms: – fever, weight loss and tiredness • Polymyalgic symptoms • Limb claudication	• Abnormal superficial temporal artery: – tender, thickened or beaded – with reduced or absent pulsation. • Scalp tenderness • Transient or permanent visual loss • Visual field defect • Relative afferent papillary defect • Anterior ischaemic optic neuritis: – pale, swollen optic disc with haemorrhages on fundoscopy. • Central retinal artery occlusion: – unilateral or bilateral. • Upper cranial nerve palsies • Features of large-vessel GCA: – asymmetry of pulses and blood pressure – bruits (usually of the upper limb)	• Herpes zoster • Migraine or other causes of headaches • Serious intracranial pathology, e.g. infiltrative retro-orbital or base of skull lesions • Other causes of acute vision loss, e.g. transient ischaemic attack • Cervical spine disease • ENT pathology, e.g. sinus, TMJ and ear disease • Systemic vasculitides • Connective tissue diseases

ENT, ear nose and throat; TMJ, temporomandibular joint.

of patients, most often at disease onset (5, 8). Transient visual loss (amaurosis fugax) occurs somewhat less frequently (10–15% of patients), but should be promptly recognized, since in nearly one-half of patients it evolves into permanent visual loss if treatment with glucocorticoids is not immediately started. Visual loss related to GCA is sudden, painless, and mostly (over 90% of patients) due to anterior ischaemic optic neuropathy (AION) caused by occlusive arteritis of posterior ciliary artery; less commonly, the retinal arteries are affected (9). Unilateral visual loss is a strong risk factor for visual loss in the contralateral eye, which occurs within a week or two in half to three-quarters of cases if glucocorticoids are not swiftly commenced (5, 10). In the odd case, posterior ischaemic optic neuropathy (PION) or occipital cortex ischaemia may be responsible for visual loss (1). Fundoscopy typically reveals a chalky white or, sometimes, an oedematous pale to pink optic disc in the early stages of AION, whereas in later stages, atrophy of the optic disc is observed (11). In contrast, disc pallor develops about 6 weeks after visual loss in PION, while fundoscopy is unremarkable in patients with cortical blindness.

Most patients that incur visual loss have other symptoms and signs indicative of GCA. However, a sizeable minority of patients may present with isolated arteritic visual loss ('occult GCA' or 'ocular GCA') (9, 12). The presence of raised inflammatory markers, suggestive funduscopic changes, and exclusion of other disorders are helpful in establishing the correct diagnosis.

4.5 Cerebrovascular ischaemic events

Cerebrovascular ischaemic events, including transient ischaemic attacks and stroke, are rarer but recognized complications of GCA. Such events are usually precocious and mostly due to vasculitis of the carotid or of the vertebrobasilar arteries (5, 13). Intracranial vasculitis leading to cerebrovascular events has been reported in patients with GCA, but only in extremely rare cases (14). In a handful of patients, angina pectoris, congestive heart failure, and myocardial infarction can be (usually early) manifestations of GCA (1). A moderately, but not very high, erythrocyte sedimentation rate and C-reactive protein at diagnosis, older age, hypertension, a past history of ischaemic heart disease, and the absence of systemic manifestations have been mapped to an increased risk of cranial ischaemic events (15–17). The development of any ischaemic complication is also associated with the risk of developing subsequent ischaemic manifestations including visual loss (17).

4.6 Constitutional symptoms

GCA can present without predominant headache or scalp tenderness and this may delay diagnosis. About half of patients with GCA have constitutional manifestations including fever, malaise, depression, anorexia, and weight loss (4). The fever is usually low grade, but it can reach 39–40°C in about 15% of cases (5). In about 15% of patients, systemic manifestations can be the only feature of GCA (18). In such cases, temporal artery biopsy (18) or imaging studies of the large vessels (19) are critical in clinching the diagnosis. Patients with marked inflammatory manifestations tend on average to incur ischaemic complications less frequently, but a strong inflammatory response by no means excludes such complications in the individual patient (6).

4.7 Large-vessel vasculitis

Up to one-quarter of patients with GCA develop clinical manifestations related to large-vessel involvement including arm claudication, arterial bruits, and heart murmurs (4, 20). Specifically, thoracic aorta aneurysms, abdominal aorta aneurysms, and large-vessel stenoses (mostly affecting the upper limb arteries) develop in 9.3%, 6.5%, and 13.5% of unselected GCA patients, respectively (21). These manifestations usually become clinically overt only 3–4 years after the onset of the symptoms of GCA. However, evidence of large-vessel involvement can be demonstrated much earlier in GCA if imaging studies of the large vessels are performed. In this regard, a sensitive technique such as ^{18}F-fluorodeoxyglucose positron emission tomography is able to reveal large-vessel vasculitis in as many as 83% of patients with early GCA (22). Other investigations such as colour Doppler sonography and magnetic resonance imaging are also able to demonstrate early large-vessel vasculitis (23).

Compared to unselected patients with GCA, those with large-vessel vasculitis have cranial symptoms less frequently and a positive temporal artery biopsy (21, 24), whereas they have an increased risk of developing aortic aneurysms and slightly higher mortality rates due to thoracic aorta dissection or rupture of aortic aneurysms (25).

4.8 Musculoskeletal symptoms and polymyalgia

Musculoskeletal symptoms and polymyalgia are quite common in patients with GCA, and may come on at any time of the disease (26). The most frequent musculoskeletal manifestation is undoubtedly PMR, which affects about 40% of patients. Other musculoskeletal manifestations are seen in approximately 25% of patients and include benign, non-erosive peripheral arthritis with or without distal swelling with pitting oedema, tenosynovitis, and carpal tunnel syndrome. Swelling with pitting oedema of the hands or feet (also known as RS3PE (remitting symmetric seronegative synovitis with pitting oedema)) due to synovitis and tenosynovitis is typically associated with PMR, although it may also be idiopathic or occur in the context of other disorders.

4.9 Cranial and peripheral neuropathies

Peripheral neuropathies complicate GCA in approximately one-sixth of patients. Both the upper and the lower limbs may be affected (4, 5). Anecdotal reports have also mapped cranial neuropathy especially oculomotor involvement (27) and plexopathy (28) to GCA. In addition, audiovestibular dysfunction manifesting as sensineural hearing loss has occasionally been observed in early GCA (29). Mild audiovestibular dysfunction may be more frequent if specifically sought for by direct questioning and specific tests (30). Glucocorticoid treatment can reverse, in full or in part, audiovestibular changes (29, 30).

Cough affects about 10% of GCA patients, presumably as a consequence of ischaemia of the cough receptors (31). Cough may be the only respiratory symptom, or be associated with sore throat and voice hoarseness (5). Other infrequent clinical manifestations of GCA include facial swelling (32), dental pain, chin numbness, glossitis, submandibular swelling (33), diplopia, Charles Bonnet syndrome (visual hallucinations probably due to ischaemia of the visual pathways), and noises in the head (such as turbine engines and tree frogs) (34). These manifestations can usually be reversed by glucocorticoids. Finally, pericardial and pleural effusions (35), female genital tract (36) and breast involvement (37), syndrome of inappropriate antidiuretic secretion (38), and dysarthria (39) have anecdotally been described as presenting features.

4.10 Physical examination

Physical examination in GCA may reveal tenderness, thickening, nodules, and occasionally reddening of the superficial temporal arteries (4, 5). Temporal artery pulses may be decreased or absent. In patients with large-vessel involvement, bruits may be heard, particularly over the arteries above the aorta (4, 5).

References

1. Hunder GG. Giant cell arteritis and polymyalgia rheumatica. *Med Clin North Am* 1997; 81:195–219.

2. Gonzalez-Gay MA, Boiardi L, Garcia-Porrua C, *et al*. Geographical and genetic factors do not account for significant differences in the clinical spectrum of giant cell arteritis in southern Europe. *J Rheumatol* 2004; 31:520–3.

3. Kobayashi S, Yano T, Matsumoto Y, et al. Clinical and epidemiologic analysis of giant cell (temporal) arteritis from a nationwide survey in 1998 in Japan: the first government-supported nationwide survey. Arthritis Rheum 2003; 49:594–8.

4. Salvarani C, Cantini F, Hunder GG. Polymyalgia rheumatica and giant-cell arteritis. Lancet 2008; 372:234–45.

5. Salvarani C, Cantini F, Boiardi L, et al. Polymyalgia rheumatica and giant-cell arteritis. N Engl J Med 2002; 347:261–71.

6. Gonzalez-Gay MA, Garcia-Porrua C, Amor-Dorado JC, et al. Fever in biopsy-proven giant cell arteritis: clinical implications in a defined population. Arthritis Rheum 2004; 51:652–5.

7. Currey J. Scalp necrosis in giant cell arteritis and review of the literature. Br J Rheumatol 1997; 36:814–16.

8. Aiello PD, Trautmann JC, McPhee TJ, et al. Visual prognosis in giant cell arteritis. Ophthalmology 1993; 100:550–5.

9. Hayreh SS, Podhajsky PA, Zimmerman B. Occult giant cell arteritis: ocular manifestations. Am J Ophthalmol 1998; 125:521–6.

10. Gordon LK, Levin LA. Visual loss in giant cell arteritis. JAMA 1998; 280:385–6.

11. Hayreh SS. Ophthalmic features of giant cell arteritis. Baillieres Clin Rheumatol 1991; 5:431–59.

12. Rahman W, Rahman FZ. Giant cell (temporal) arteritis: an overview and update. Surv Ophthalmol 2005; 50:415–28.

13. Ruegg S, Engelter S, Jeanneret C, et al. Bilateral vertebral artery occlusion resulting from giant cell arteritis: report of 3 cases and review of the literature. Medicine (Baltimore) 2003; 82:1–12.

14. Salvarani C, Giannini C, Miller DV, et al. Giant cell arteritis: involvement of intracranial arteries. Arthritis Rheum 2006; 55:985–9.

15. Salvarani C, Della Bella BC, Cimino L, et al. Risk factors for severe cranial ischaemic events in an Italian population-based cohort of patients with giant cell arteritis. Rheumatology (Oxford) 2009; 48:250–3.

16. Hernandez-Rodriguez J, Garcia-Martinez A, Casademont J, et al. A strong initial systemic inflammatory response is associated with higher corticosteroid requirements and longer duration of therapy in patients with giant-cell arteritis. Arthritis Rheum 2002; 47:29–35.

17. Salvarani C, Cimino L, Macchioni P, et al. Risk factors for visual loss in an Italian population-based cohort of patients with giant cell arteritis. Arthritis Rheum 2005; 53:293–7.

18. Calamia KT, Hunder GG. Giant cell arteritis (temporal arteritis) presenting as fever of undetermined origin. Arthritis Rheum 1981; 24:1414–18.

19. Meller J, Strutz F, Siefker U, et al. Early diagnosis and follow-up of aortitis with ((18)F)FDG PET and MRI. Eur J Nucl Med Mol Imaging 2003; 30:730–6.

20. Nuenninghoff DM, Hunder GG, Christianson TJ, et al. Incidence and predictors of large-artery complication (aortic aneurysm, aortic dissection, and/or large-artery stenosis) in patients with giant cell arteritis: a population-based study over 50 years. Arthritis Rheum 2003; 48:3522–31.

21. Bongartz T, Matteson EL. Large-vessel involvement in giant cell arteritis. Curr Opin Rheumatol 2006; 18:10–17.

22. Blockmans D, De Ceuninck L, Vanderschueren S, et al. Repetitive 18F-fluorodeoxyglucose positron emission tomography in giant cell arteritis: a prospective study of 35 patients. Arthritis Rheum 2006; 55:131–7.

23. Pipitone N, Versari A, Salvarani C. Role of imaging studies in the diagnosis and follow-up of large-vessel vasculitis: an update. Rheumatology (Oxford) 2008; 47:403–8.

24. Brack A, Martinez-Taboada V, Stanson A, et al. Disease pattern in cranial and large-vessel giant cell arteritis. Arthritis Rheum 1999; 42:311–17.

25. Nuenninghoff DM, Hunder GG, Christianson TJ, *et al*. Mortality of large-artery complication (aortic aneurysm, aortic dissection, and/or large-artery stenosis) in patients with giant cell arteritis: a population-based study over 50 years. *Arthritis Rheum* 2003; 48:3532–7.

26. Salvarani C, Hunder GG. Musculoskeletal manifestations in a population-based cohort of patients with giant cell arteritis. *Arthritis Rheum* 1999; 42:1259–66.

27. Loffredo L, Parrotto S, Violi F. Giant cell arteritis, oculomotor nerve palsy, and acute hearing loss. *Scand J Rheumatol* 2004; 33:279–80.

28. Gatfosse M, Santin A, Chamouard JM. Giant cell arteritis revealed by bilateral lesions of brachial plexus. *Rev Rhum Engl Ed* 1996; 63:301–2.

29. Hausch RC, Harrington T. Temporal arteritis and sensorineural hearing loss. *Semin Arthritis Rheum* 1998; 28:206–9.

30. Amor-Dorado JC, Llorca J, Garcia-Porrua C, *et al*. Audiovestibular manifestations in giant cell arteritis: a prospective study. *Medicine (Baltimore)* 2003; 82:13–26.

31. Olopade CO, Sekosan M, Schraufnagel DE. Giant cell arteritis manifesting as chronic cough and fever of unknown origin. *Mayo Clin Proc* 1997; 72:1048–50.

32. Liozon E, Ouattara B, Portal MF, *et al*. Head-and-neck swelling: an under-recognized feature of giant cell arteritis. A report of 37 patients. *Clin Exp Rheumatol* 2006; 24:S20–S25.

33. Porter MJ. Temporal arteritis presenting as a submandibular swelling. *J Laryngol Otol* 1990; 104:819–20.

34. Stone JH. Vasculitis: a collection of pearls and myths. *Rheum Dis Clin North Am* 2007; 33:691–739.

35. Valstar MH, Terpstra WF, de Jong RS. Pericardial and pleural effusion in giant cell arteritis. *Am J Med* 2003; 114:708–9.

36. Bajocchi G, Zamorani G, Cavazza A, *et al*. Giant-cell arteritis of the female genital tract associated with occult temporal arteritis and FDG-PET evidence of large-vessel vasculitis. *Clin Exp Rheumatol* 2007; 25:S36–S39.

37. Kariv R, Sidi Y, Gur H. Systemic vasculitis presenting as a tumorlike lesion. Four case reports and an analysis of 79 reported cases. *Medicine (Baltimore)* 2000; 79:349–59.

38. Luzar MJ, Whisler RL, Hunder GG. Syndrome of inappropriate antidiuretic hormone secretion in association with temporal arteritis. *J Rheumatol* 1982; 9:957–60.

39. Lee CC, Su WW, Hunder GG. Dysarthria associated with giant cell arteritis. *J Rheumatol* 1999; 26:931–2.

Part 2

Diagnostic work-up

5	Laboratory findings	43
6	Ultrasound	49
7	Temporal artery biopsy	59
8	Positron emission tomography and magnetic resonance imaging	63
9	Differential diagnosis	73

Chapter 5

Laboratory findings

Nicolò Pipitone

Key points

- There are no specific blood tests for polymyalgia rheumatica (PMR) and giant cell arteritis (GCA). However, it is important to document a basic laboratory dataset to exclude mimics such as cancer, infection, inflammatory arthritis vasculitis, and connective tissue diseases.
- Autoimmunity serology is negative in PMR and GCA.
- It is unusual for patients with PMR and GCA to have normal erythrocyte sedimentation rate and C-reactive protein values.

5.1 Laboratory findings in polymyalgia rheumatica and giant cell arteritis

The 2015 European League Against Rheumatism and American College of Rheumatology recommendations for PMR suggest that there should be documentation of a basic laboratory dataset prior to the prescription of glucocorticoids in every case of PMR. The objective is to exclude mimicking conditions and establish a baseline for monitoring of therapy. The tests should include rheumatoid factor and/or anticyclic citrullinated peptide antibodies (ACPAs), C-reactive protein (CRP) and/or erythrocyte sedimentation rate (ESR), blood count, glucose, creatinine, liver function tests, bone profile (including calcium and alkaline phosphatase), and dipstick urinalysis. Additional investigations to consider are protein electrophoresis, thyroid stimulating hormone, creatine kinase, and vitamin D.

Depending on clinical signs and symptoms and the likelihood of the alternative diagnoses, additional more extensive serological tests such as antinuclear antibodies (ANAs), antineutrophil cytoplasmic antibodies (ANCAs), or tuberculosis tests may be performed to exclude mimicking conditions. Additional investigations such as chest radiographs may be considered at the discretion of the physician in order to exclude other diagnoses.

Laboratory findings in PMR and GCA themselves, are non-specific and reflect systemic inflammation. Traditionally, an elevated ESR is considered the hallmark of both disorders. An ESR of at least 30 mm/1st hour is included in most diagnostic and classification criteria for PMR (1), while an ESR of 50 mm/1st hour or greater is one of the American College of Rheumatology criteria for classifying patients as having GCA (2). Approximately 6–7% of patients with PMR have lower (< 40 mm/1st hour) ESR values

(3, 4). Similarly, an ESR less than 50 mm/1st hour and less than 40 mm/1st hour has been noted in 5% and 11% of patients with GCA, respectively (5).

CRP is a more sensitive inflammatory marker than ESR. It is also more specific to inflammation than ESR, which may be influenced by age, gender, anaemia, and levels of various plasma proteins (6). In PMR, a normal CRP has been recorded in 1% of cases (versus 6% of cases with a normal ESR) (3), while in biopsy-proven GCA, the sensitivity of the CRP is about 87–98% compared with a sensitivity of about 80–84%% of the ESR (7). Only a very small number (~ 4%) of patients with GCA have both ESR and CRP in the normal range at presentation prior to the onset of glucocorticoid therapy (8). In PMR, lower inflammatory markers are associated with male gender and less intense systemic manifestations (3, 4). Likewise, patients with GCA who have lower ESR values tend to have less frequent systemic manifestations (5). A few reports suggest that lack of high ESR/CRP values at diagnosis are also risk factors for cranial ischaemic complications in patients with GCA (9). However, according to current knowledge, neither the ESR nor the CRP values are helpful in predicting the risk of GCA-related ischaemic complications such as visual loss in the individual patient (5, 10, 11).

In addition to the ESR and CRP, other laboratory parameters often reflect the inflammatory status. In particular, a high fibrinogen (there are reports that it may be less sensitive but more specific than ESR) (12–14), raised alpha-2 globulins (15, 16), (usually mild) thrombocytosis (17, 18), low albumin (18), increased complement levels (19), and anaemia of the chronic inflammatory type (18) can all occur in variable combinations both in PMR and GCA.

Serum interleukin 6 (IL-6) is one of the most sensitive indices of disease activity, but it is not measured in routine clinical practice (20). However, there are reports suggesting a role for it as a biomarker for subclinical disease activity as well as a biomarker predicting risk of flares.

Liver enzymes, particularly alkaline phosphatase, are raised in approximately one-quarter to one-third of patients (18, 21). The elevation is usually modest and returns to normal after treatment (18). Renal function tests are mostly normal, although very rarely microscopic haematuria and minimal proteinuria responsive to glucocorticoid therapy can occur. Nephrotic-range proteinuria is exceptional, but should alert to an underlying secondary amyloidosis (22). Occasionally, thyroid function tests may be abnormal (23).

Autoantibodies, including ANAs, rheumatoid factor, ACPAs, and ANCAs are typically negative (1, 19). These autoantibodies may serve as important tests to exclude late-onset polymyalgic inflammatory arthritis, connective tissue diseases, and vasculitides, especially in the context of severe constitutional symptoms, very high inflammatory markers, and poor response to glucocorticoids. Nevertheless, it should be borne in mind that in approximately 10% of elderly subjects the rheumatoid factor and ANA may be non-specifically positive, usually at low titre (24). In contrast, ACPAs are more specific to rheumatoid arthritis, and their presence should prompt considerations for a PMR-like elderly-onset rheumatoid arthritis. In the few patients that test positive for ANCA, antiproteinase-3 (anti-PR3) and antimyeloperoxidase antibodies are negative. Positive anti-PR3 requires exclusion of an underlying vasculitis with a polymyalgic onset (19). Creatine kinase and other muscle enzymes are typically normal in PMR despite muscle aching (19).

Up to one-half of untreated patients with active GCA may test positive tests for anticardiolipin antibodies, but anticardiolipin antibodies can be seen non-specifically in other situations such as infection and do not increase the risk of thrombotic events in GCA. However, anticardiolipin antibodies correlate, at least to some extent, with

GCA activity, and normalize as a rule after treatment onset (25, 26). Immunoglobulin G against the human ferritin heavy chain has been found in 73–92% of patients with untreated GCA, but the sensitivity drops dramatically in patients in remission (27, 28).

Measurements of inflammatory markers are usually repeated over time to monitor disease activity and gauge response to treatment in PMR and GCA. Flares of PMR and GCA are often heralded by an increase in inflammatory indices (29). However, an isolated elevation of inflammatory markers should not be treated as a disease flare in the absence of symptoms (1). Frequent monitoring checks of ESR or CRP is also unnecessary in the stable patient. A possible exception is ocular GCA (GCA affecting the eye only), where monitoring of inflammatory markers is the only way to assess disease activity. The CRP (and, where available, IL-6) are probably superior to the ESR in assessing disease activity since the ESR can be abnormal for reasons unrelated to inflammation (6). Occasionally, failure to adequately suppress the inflammatory response with adequate glucocorticoid doses in a patient with PMR may suggest an underlying arteritis (19).

Finally, because IL-6 is a key stimulator of serum inflammatory markers, including the ESR and CRP, it is unclear how reliably such markers effectively reflect inflammation in patients treated with inhibitors of the IL-6 pathway (30).

Soluble biomarkers may hold promise in identifying patients with GCA and perhaps those patients that have an increased risk of developing ischaemic complications. Pentraxin 3 (PTX3), which is structurally related to CRP and serum amyloid A but is made by endothelial cells and activated leucocytes, is one of the most promising markers reported to date (31). Elevated circulating levels of PTX3 have been linked to recent onset of GCA or optic nerve ischaemia; optic nerve ischaemia has also been shown to correlate with increased circulating vascular endothelial growth factor levels (32). Other potential markers of interest include neutrophil surface molecules such as annexin A1 (33) as well as markers of the T-helper-1/T-helper-17 axis (34).

References

1. Salvarani C, Cantini F, Boiardi L, et al. Polymyalgia rheumatica and giant-cell arteritis. N Engl J Med 2002; 347:261–71.

2. Hunder GG, Bloch DA, Michel BA, et al. The American College of Rheumatology 1990 criteria for the classification of giant cell arteritis. Arthritis Rheum 1990; 33:1122–8.

3. Cantini F, Salvarani C, Olivieri I, et al. Erythrocyte sedimentation rate and C-reactive protein in the evaluation of disease activity and severity in polymyalgia rheumatica: a prospective follow-up study. Semin Arthritis Rheum 2000; 30:17–24.

4. Proven A, Gabriel SE, O'Fallon WM, et al. Polymyalgia rheumatica with low erythrocyte sedimentation rate at diagnosis. J Rheumatol 1999; 26:1333–7.

5. Salvarani C, Hunder GG. Giant cell arteritis with low erythrocyte sedimentation rate: frequency of occurrence in a population-based study. Arthritis Rheum 2001; 45:140–5.

6. Salvarani C, Cantini F, Boiardi L, et al. Laboratory investigations useful in giant cell arteritis and Takayasu's arteritis. Clin Exp Rheumatol 2003; 21:S23–S28.

7. Parikh M, Miller NR, Lee AG, et al. Prevalence of a normal C-reactive protein with an elevated erythrocyte sedimentation rate in biopsy-proven giant cell arteritis. Ophthalmology 2006; 113:1842–5.

8. Kermani TA, Schmidt J, Crowson CS, et al. Utility of erythrocyte sedimentation rate and C-reactive protein for the diagnosis of giant cell arteritis. Semin Arthritis Rheum 2012; 41:866–71.

9. Salvarani C, Della BC, Cimino L, *et al.* Risk factors for severe cranial ischaemic events in an Italian population-based cohort of patients with giant cell arteritis. *Rheumatology (Oxford)* 2009; 48:250–3.

10. Schmidt D, Vaith P. Acute-phase response and the risk of developing ischemic complications in giant cell arteritis: comment on the article by Cid et al. *Arthritis Rheum* 2000; 43:234–6.

11. Cid MC, Font C, Oristrell J, *et al.* Association between strong inflammatory response and low risk of developing visual loss and other cranial ischemic complications in giant cell (temporal) arteritis. *Arthritis Rheum* 1998; 41:26–32.

12. McCarthy EM, MacMullan PA, Al-Mudhaffer S, *et al.* Plasma fibrinogen is an accurate marker of disease activity in patients with polymyalgia rheumatica. *Rheumatology (Oxford)* 2013; 52(3):465–71.

13. Schreiber S, Buyse M. The CRP initial response to treatment as prognostic factor in patients with polymyalgia rheumatica. *Clin Rheumatol* 1995; 14:315–18.

14. Gudmundsson M, Nordborg E, Bengtsson BA, *et al.* Plasma viscosity in giant cell arteritis as a predictor of disease activity. *Ann Rheum Dis* 1993; 52:104–9.

15. Gilbert GJ. Diagnosing temporal arteritis. *JAMA* 2002; 288:1352–3.

16. Subrahmanyam P, Dasgupta B. Polymyalgia rheumatica. *Medicine (Baltimore)* 2006; 34:427–30.

17. Foroozan R, Danesh-Meyer H, Savino PJ, *et al.* Thrombocytosis in patients with biopsy-proven giant cell arteritis. *Ophthalmology* 2002; 109:1267–71.

18. Kyle V. Laboratory investigations including liver in polymyalgia rheumatica/giant cell arteritis. *Baillieres Clin Rheumatol* 1991; 5:475–84.

19. Hunder GG. Giant cell arteritis and polymyalgia rheumatica. *Med Clin North Am* 1997; 81:195–219.

20. Salvarani C, Cantini F, Hunder GG. Polymyalgia rheumatica and giant-cell arteritis. *Lancet* 2008; 372:234–45.

21. Kyle V, Wraight EP, Hazleman BL. Liver scan abnormalities in polymyalgia rheumatica/giant cell arteritis. *Clin Rheumatol* 1991; 10:294–7.

22. Monteagudo M, Vidal G, Andreu J, *et al.* Giant cell (temporal) arteritis and secondary renal amyloidosis: report of 2 cases. *J Rheumatol* 1997; 24:605–7.

23. Weyand CM, Goronzy JJ. Medium- and large-vessel vasculitis. *N Engl J Med* 2003; 349:160–9.

24. Lopez-Hoyos M, Ruiz de Alegria A, Blanco R, *et al.* Clinical utility of anti-CCP antibodies in the differential diagnosis of elderly-onset rheumatoid arthritis and polymyalgia rheumatica. *Rheumatology (Oxford)* 2004; 43:655–7.

25. Liozon E, Roblot P, Paire D, *et al.* Anticardiolipin antibody levels predict flares and relapses in patients with giant-cell (temporal) arteritis. A longitudinal study of 58 biopsy-proven cases. *Rheumatology (Oxford)* 2000; 39:1089–94.

26. Nakaoka Y, Higuchi K, Arita Y, *et al.* Tocilizumab for the treatment of patients with refractory Takayasu arteritis. *Int Heart J* 2013; 54:405–11.

27. Baerlecken NT, Linnemann A, Gross WL, *et al.* Association of ferritin autoantibodies with giant cell arteritis/polymyalgia rheumatica. *Ann Rheum Dis* 2012; 71(6):943–7.

28. Régent A, Ly KH, Blet A, *et al.* Contribution of antiferritin antibodies to diagnosis of giant cell arteritis. *Ann Rheum Dis* 2013; 72(7):1269–70.

29. Kyle V, Cawston TE, Hazleman BL. Erythrocyte sedimentation rate and C reactive protein in the assessment of polymyalgia rheumatica/giant cell arteritis on presentation and during follow up. *Ann Rheum Dis* 1989; 48:667–71.

30. Bredemeier M, Rocha CM, Barbosa MV, *et al.* One-year clinical and radiological evolution of a patient with refractory Takayasu's arteritis under treatment with tocilizumab. *Clin Exp Rheumatol* 2012; 30:S98–100.

31. Monach PA. Biomarkers in vasculitis. *Curr Opin Rheumatol* 2014; 26(1):24–30.

32. Baldini M, Maugeri N, Ramirez GA, *et al*. Selective up-regulation of the soluble pattern-recognition receptor PTX3 and of vascular endothelial growth factor in giant cell arteritis: relevance for recent optic nerve ischemia. *Arthritis Rheum* 2012; 64(3):854–65.

33. Nadkarni S, Dalli J, Hollywood J, *et al*. Investigational analysis reveals a potential role for neutrophils in giant-cell arteritis disease progression. *Circ Res* 2014; 114(2):242–8.

34. Samson M, Audia S, Fraszczak J, *et al*. Th1 and Th17 lymphocytes expressing CD161 are implicated in giant cell arteritis and polymyalgia rheumatica pathogenesis. *Arthritis Rheum* 2012; 64(11):3788–98.

Chapter 6

Ultrasound

Wolfgang A. Schmidt

Key points

- Ultrasound helps to differentiate polymyalgia rheumatica (PMR) from other diseases with similar symptoms by detecting subdeltoid bursitis, biceps tenosynovitis, glenohumeral and hip joint effusions, as well as trochanteric bursitis.

- Ultrasound of temporal and axillary arteries detects giant cell arteritis (GCA) in about 15% of patients with pure PMR.

- Fast-track clinics offering appointments within 24 hours for patients with suspected PMR or GCA provide history, clinical examination, and ultrasound by a specialist and may help early diagnosis and prevention of sight loss.

6.1 Introduction

Ultrasound is widely available in rheumatology practice (1, 2). Image quality and spatial resolution has dramatically increased in the last years. This allows detection of characteristic vascular and musculoskeletal pathology in GCA and PMR (3, 4). Ideally, ultrasound is part of history taking and clinical examination where diagnosis is quickly established or excluded, and specific treatment is planned in the same session. Time elapsed during the examination can be utilized by the experienced sonographer to interact with the patient for further details of history, clinical findings, and explanation of the diagnosis and treatment. Ultrasound is non-invasive, well tolerated by patients, and easily repeatable. Findings can be documented as still images or videos. Videos of temporal artery pathology in particular allow confirmation of findings by external reviewers.

6.2 Ultrasound in polymyalgia rheumatica

Ultrasound of the shoulder and hip regions often reveals characteristic pathologies in PMR (Table 6.1; Figures 6.1) (5–8).

Shoulder and hip ultrasound has been incorporated into the European League Against Rheumatism/American College of Rheumatology (EULAR/ACR) provisional classification criteria (9). An algorithm that includes shoulder and hip ultrasound exhibits a higher specificity in comparison to an algorithm without ultrasound. It has been

Table 6.1 Characteristic ultrasound findings in PMR

Anatomical region	Pathology	Definition
Shoulder	Subdeltoid bursitis (Figure 6.2)	Fluid with a sagittal diameter of >2 mm between rotator cuff and deltoid muscle (5)
Shoulder	Tenosynovitis of the long biceps tendon (Figure 6.3)	Abnormal hypoechoic or anechoic thickened tissue within the tendon sheath (6)
Shoulder	Glenohumeral joint effusion	Abnormal fluid in the posterior joint region (> 3 mm) particularly with external rotation, or in the axillary recess (> 3.7 mm) (7)
Hip	Hip joint effusion	Abnormal fluid in the anterior femoral recess (> 8 mm distance between bone and anterior rim of capsule) (5)
Hip	Trochanteric bursitis	Abnormal fluid between gluteus medius tendon and surrounding muscles (8)

shown that the EULAR/ACR algorithm that includes ultrasound exhibits the best ratio between positive and negative predictive value when compared with all relevant other diagnostic or classification criteria, particularly because of its high specificity (10). PMR patients in whom ultrasound revealed inflammation in the shoulder and hip region respond better to glucocorticoid treatment (11).

Other bursitides around the hip joint such as iliopsoas bursitis are less frequently detected by ultrasound in PMR. Knee joint effusions frequently occur in PMR (12).

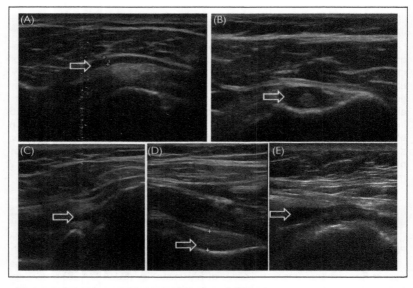

Figure 6.1 Ultrasound findings in PMR indicated by the arrows: (A) subdeltoid bursitis; (B) tenosynovitis of the biceps tendon; (C) effusion of the glenohumeral joint; (D) effusion of the hip joint; (E) trochanteric bursitis.

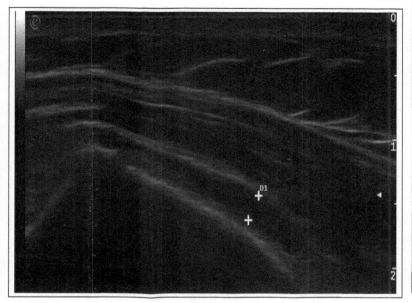

Figure 6.2 Ultrasound findings in PMR, unilateral subacromial subdeltoid bursitis in PMR.

6.3 Ultrasound is particularly important to rule out other diseases that may mimic polymyalgia rheumatica

- Shoulder or hip osteoarthritis showing diffuse irregularities of the humeral or femoral bone surface
- Rotator cuff pathologies such as tendinitis (thickened heterogeneous tendons) calcifying tendinitis (hyperechoic lesions in the rotator cuff), and rotator cuff tears

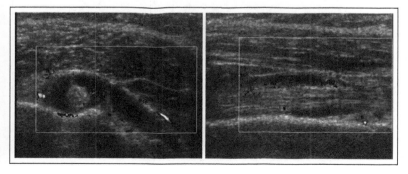

Figure 6.3 (See colour plate section). Shoulder ultrasound findings in PMR, bilateral TS biceps tendon.

- Rheumatoid arthritis (Figure 6.4) with often larger effusions and bursitides, erosions of the humeral head, detection of synovitis in joints that are not involved in PMR, such as metacarpophalangeal or metatarsophalangeal joints
- Pain syndrome with normal anatomical appearance of shoulders and hips.

A subgroup of PMR patients show features of GCA or large-vessel vasculitis. In 7% of patients with PMR but no symptoms of temporal arteritis, temporal artery ultrasound

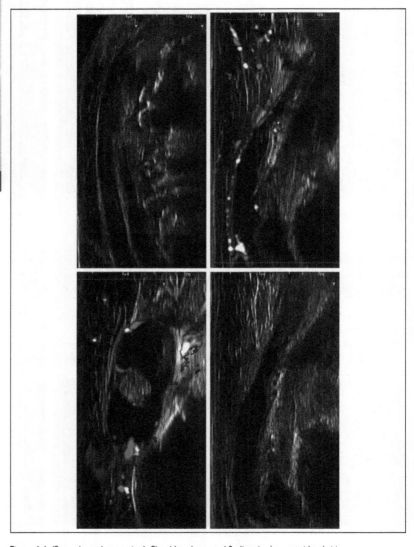

Figure 6.4 (See colour plate section). Shoulder ultrasound findings in rheumatoid arthritis.

was positive (13). Adding ultrasound of axillary arteries will detect GCA in about 15% of patients with 'pure PMR' (4).

6.4 **Ultrasound in temporal arteritis**

Ultrasound shows a circumferential hypoechoic wall thickening in active temporal arteritis (Figure 6.5). This phenomenon has been called the 'halo sign' (14). It is hypoechoic (dark), not anechoic (black), and it represents oedematous inflammatory tissue of the artery wall. This tissue is not compressible (15). In addition, stenoses may occur in which colour Doppler shows a blurring mixture of colours (aliasing) together with persistent diastolic blood flow. Pulsed wave Doppler displays an at least twofold increase of the maximum systolic blood flow velocity in the stenosis compared to a segment before or behind the stenosis. Temporal arteries may occlude with ultrasound and may not display intravascular colour Doppler signals.

The temporal artery halo sign usually disappears after 2–3 weeks with glucocorticoid treatment (14). In some patients, ultrasound diagnosis already becomes more difficult after a few days (16) while a few patients may exhibit some wall pathology for a few months (17). Figure 6.6A shows the anatomy of the superficial temporal artery with its frontal and parietal branches.

The sonographer should have examined temporal arteries of about 30–50 healthy subjects and should have seen at least three to five patients with definite temporal arteritis before using this method for routine practice. Temporal artery ultrasound includes bilateral longitudinal and transverse scans of the common superficial temporal arteries and of the frontal and parietal branches.

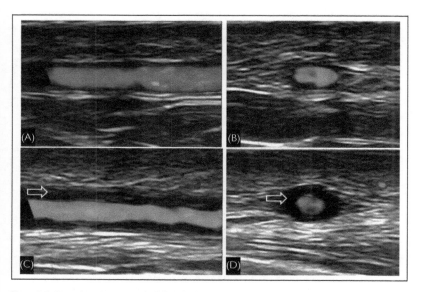

Figure 6.5 (See colour plate section). Colour Doppler ultrasound image of temporal arteries. Longitudinal and transverse scans of a normal temporal artery (A, B), and in temporal arteritis showing hypoechoic wall thickening (arrows) (C, D).

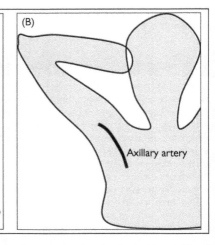

Figure 6.6 Anatomy of the common superficial temporal artery with its frontal and parietal branch (A) and the axillary artery (B).

The technical requirements for temporal artery ultrasound are as follows:

- Modern, high-quality ultrasound equipment
- Linear ultrasound probe
- The probe should have a frequency of at least 10 MHz for greyscale ultrasound, preferably 15 MHz or more, leading to a resolution of about 0.1–0.2 mm, and greater than 7 MHz for colour Doppler ultrasound.

Pitfalls for temporal artery ultrasound are listed in Table 6.2.

Table 6.2 Pitfalls for temporal artery ultrasound		
Pitfall	Reason	Solution
Colour filling only the centre of the artery lumen	Colour gain too low PRF[a] too high No colour box steering	Adjust colour gain in healthy subject PRF should be 2–3 kHz Angle between ultrasound beam and artery should be > 60°
No colour flow visible	Pressure on probe too high Hair inhibits visibility	Release pressure on probe More ultrasound gel, slightly increase pressure on probe
Colour spills over the artery wall	Colour gain too high PRF[a] too low	Decrease colour gain Use same settings in each patient
Halo cannot be distinguished from lumen in B-mode image	B-gain too low Not enough contrast	Increase B-gain Decrease dynamic range
No halo seen	Incomplete scan Resolved with treatment	All segments should be examined See patients as early as possible Examine also axillary arteries
[a] Pulse repetition frequency.		

Several studies and three meta-analyses have evaluated the diagnostic performance of temporal artery ultrasound (18–20). Ultrasound performs well particularly with well-trained sonographers in specialized centres using high-end ultrasound technology reaching sensitivities and particularly specificities of well over 90% compared to the clinical diagnosis of GCA. Multicentre studies like the international TABUL (Temporal Artery Biopsy versus Ultrasound) study show that stored videos provide comprehensive documentation of pathology.

As the temporal artery wall swelling disappears quickly and reoccurs only in more severe flares, patients should be seen as early as possible. Fast-track clinics have been implemented in specialized centres for which patients receive an appointment within 24 hours (3, 4, 21, 22). Diagnosis can be quickly established with clinical examination and ultrasound by either one experienced rheumatologist of a team of specialists. Early diagnosis and treatment has been shown to prevent sight loss.

Other cranial arteries can also be examined by ultrasound. The occipital arteries may be involved in patients presenting with retroauricular pain, and the facial arteries particularly in patients with jaw claudication.

6.5 Ultrasound in large-vessel giant cell arteritis

Extracranial arterial involvement in GCA is more common than previously assumed. About 50% of newly diagnosed GCA patients exhibit vasculitis of the axillary arteries (23). Adding axillary ultrasound to temporal artery ultrasound increases the diagnostic yield for GCA, particularly as only 60% of patients with large-vessel GCA have temporal artery involvement. A sonographer examining both the temporal and axillary arteries should identify more GCA patients than biopsy with histology of a 1–2 cm long segment of the temporal artery (3).

The axillary and proximal brachial arteries can be easily and quickly examined with ultrasound. Figure 6.6B shows the anatomy of the axillary artery. The probe is placed longitudinally in the axilla along the humeral head and neck. This scan is identical with the axillary shoulder scan for detecting glenohumeral joint effusions. The axillary artery localizes either at the level of the humerus or 1–2 cm medially to it. It is sufficient to examine the axillary artery and the contiguous first 10 cm of the brachial artery. Findings are confirmed with transverse scans.

In order to receive a good colour Doppler image the colour box needs to be steered as described earlier, in order to avoid a blood flow perpendicular to the sound waves. For evaluating the artery wall with the greyscale image, the probe and vessel should be parallel. The intima–media complex of a normal axillary artery is below 1.0 mm. A bright line represents the interface between artery lumen and vessel wall followed by a dark line representing wall tissue and another bright line representing the interface between media and adventitia.

In case of vasculitis, the artery wall is thickened, usually more than 1 mm (Figure 6.7). A homogeneous wall swelling, preferably circumferential, of 1.5 mm or more is pathognomonic for axillary vasculitis (23). Vasculitis may lead to stenosis showing aliasing and characteristic pulsed wave Doppler curves with increased systolic and diastolic flow velocities as previously explained. Sometimes these arteries may occlude because of vasculitis.

The subclavian, common carotid, and vertebral arteries can also be examined in the search for vasculitis. The femoral and popliteal arteries may be examined if pedal pulses are absent (24). In GCA, the other arteries are most commonly affected only if

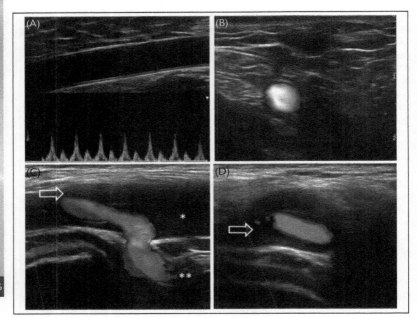

Figure 6.7 (See colour plate section). Ultrasound in large-vessel GCA: (A) longitudinal scan of a normal axillary artery (B-mode image and pulsed wave Doppler flow curves); (B) colour Doppler ultrasound transverse scan of a normal axillary artery; (C) longitudinal axillary artery scan in large-vessel GCA showing hypoechoic wall thickening of the axillary artery (arrow), occlusion of the proximal brachial artery (*) and collateral flow in the circumflexa humeri artery (**); blue colour indicates blood flow away from the probe; and (D) transverse axillary artery scan in GCA.

temporal and/or axillary arteries are involved. Vasculitic stenoses and occlusions may occur in the vertebral arteries causing cerebral ischaemia and stroke (25).

Arteriosclerosis is uncommon in the temporal and axillary arteries. It is hyperechoic, inhomogeneous, and often asymmetric. The aorta and the carotid, femoral, and popliteal arteries are much more often affected by arteriosclerosis. Occasionally, it is difficult to differentiate hypoechoic plaques from vasculitic lesions.

Ultrasound may be performed every 6 months for follow-up in order to measure the maximum wall thickness and monitor response to therapy (26). If the diameter decreases or remains the same, it is likely that the disease is controlled although rigorous prospective longitudinal studies are required.

In conclusion, ultrasound has become a valuable diagnostic tool for GCA and PMR. It aids in establishing a clear diagnosis. Fast-track clinics involving medical history, clinical examination, and ultrasound by experts may even help prevent complications such as blindness.

References

1. Schmidt WA. Ultrasound in rheumatology. *Int J Rheum Dis* 2014; 17:711–15.

2. Bruyn GA, Schmidt WA. *Introductory Guide to Musculoskeletal Ultrasound for the Rheumatologist.* Houten: Bohn Stafleu van Loghum/Springer, 2011.

3. Schmidt WA. Ultrasound in vasculitis. *Clin Exp Rheumatol* 2014; 32(1 Suppl 80):S71–7.

4. Schmidt WA. Role of ultrasound in the understanding and management of vasculitis. *Ther Adv Musculoskelet Dis* 2014; 6:39–47.

5. Schmidt WA, Schmidt H, Schicke B, *et al*. Standard reference values for musculoskeletal ultrasonography. *Ann Rheum Dis* 2004; 63:988–94.

6. Wakefield RJ, Balint PV, Szkudlarek M, *et al*. Musculoskeletal ultrasound including definitions for ultrasonographic pathology. *J Rheumatol* 2005; 32:2485–7.

7. Schmidt WA, Schicke B, Krause A. Which ultrasound scan is the best to detect glenohumeral joint effusions? *Ultraschall Med* 2008 (Suppl 5):250–5.

8. Cantini F, Niccoli L, Nannini C, *et al*. Inflammatory changes of hip synovial structures in polymyalgia rheumatica. *Clin Exp Rheumatol* 2005; 23:462–8.

9. Dasgupta B, Cimmino MA, Maradit-Kremers H, *et al*. 2012 provisional classification criteria for polymyalgia rheumatica: a European League Against Rheumatism/American College of Rheumatology collaborative initiative. *Ann Rheum Dis* 2012; 71:484–92.

10. Macchioni P, Boiardi L, Catanoso M, *et al*. Performance of the new 2012 EULAR/ACR classification criteria for polymyalgia rheumatica: comparison with the previous criteria in a single-centre study. *Ann Rheum Dis* 2014; 73:1190–3.

11. Matteson EL, Maradit-Kremers H, Cimmino MA, *et al*. Patient-reported outcomes in polymyalgia rheumatica. *J Rheumatol* 2012; 39: 795–803.

12. Cimmino MA, Camellino D, Paparo F, *et al*. High frequency of capsular knee involvement in polymyalgia rheumatica/giant cell arteritis patients studied by positron emission tomography. *Rheumatology (Oxford)* 2013; 52:1865–72.

13. Schmidt WA, Gromnica-Ihle E. Incidence of temporal arteritis in patients with polymyalgia rheumatica: a prospective study using colour Doppler sonography of the temporal arteries. *Rheumatology (Oxford)* 2002; 41:46–52.

14. Schmidt WA, Kraft HE, Vorpahl K, *et al*. Color duplex ultrasonography in the diagnosis of temporal arteritis. *N Engl J Med* 1997; 337:1336–42.

15. Aschwanden M, Daikeler T, Kesten F, *et al*. Temporal artery compression sign – a novel ultrasound finding for the diagnosis of giant cell arteritis. *Ultraschall Med* 2013; 34:47–50.

16. Hauenstein C, Reinhard M, Geiger J, *et al*. Effects of early corticosteroid treatment on magnetic resonance imaging and ultrasonography findings in giant cell arteritis. *Rheumatology (Oxford)* 2012; 51:1999–2003.

17. De Miguel E, Roxo A, Castillo C, *et al*. The utility and sensitivity of colour Doppler ultrasound in monitoring changes in giant cell arteritis. *Clin Exp Rheumatol* 2012; 30(1 Suppl 70):S34–8.

18. Karassa FB, Matsagas MI, Schmidt WA, *et al*. Diagnostic performance of ultrasonography for giant-cell arteritis: a meta-analysis. *Ann Intern Med* 2005; 142:359–69.

19. Arida A, Kyprianou M, Kanakis M, *et al*. The diagnostic value of ultrasonography-derived edema of the temporal artery wall in giant cell arteritis: a second meta-analysis. *BMC Musculoskeletal Disord* 2010; 11:44.

20. Ball EL, Walsh SR, Tang TY, *et al*. Role of ultrasonography in the diagnosis of temporal arteritis. *Br J Surg* 2010; 97:1765–71.

21. Patil P, Achilleos K, Williams M, *et al*. Outcomes and cost effectiveness analysis of fast track pathway in giant cell arteritis. *Rheumatology (Oxford)* 2014; 53 (Suppl 2):i5–6.

22. Diamantopoulos AP, Haugeberg G, Lindland A, *et al*. The fast-track ultrasound clinic for early diagnosis of giant cell arteritis significantly reduces permanent visual impairment: Towards a more effective strategy to improve clinical outcome in giant cell arteritis. *Rheumatology (Oxford)*. First published online: August 18, 2015. doi: 10.1093/rheumatology/kev289

23. Schmidt WA, Seifert A, Gromnica-Ihle E, *et al*. Ultrasound of proximal upper extremity arteries to increase the diagnostic yield in large-vessel giant cell arteritis. *Rheumatology (Oxford)* 2008; 47:96–101.

24. Czihal M, Tatò F, Rademacher A, *et al*. Involvement of the femoropopliteal arteries in giant cell arteritis: clinical and color duplex sonography. *J Rheumatol* 2012; 39:314–21.

25. García-García J, Ayo-Martín Ó, Argandoña-Palacios L, *et al*. Vertebral artery halo sign in patients with stroke: a key clue for the prompt diagnosis of giant cell arteritis. *Stroke* 2011; 42:3287–90.

26. Schmidt WA, Moll A, Seifert A, *et al*. Prognosis of large-vessel giant cell arteritis. *Rheumatology (Oxford)* 2008; 47:1406–8.

Chapter 7

Temporal artery biopsy

Francesco Muratore and Nicolò Pipitone

Key points

- Temporal artery biopsy (TAB) remains the gold standard to diagnose giant cell arteritis (GCA).
- A negative TAB does not rule out GCA.
- In a minority of patients, histological inflammation may be confined to the adventitial or periarterial small vessels.

7.1 Temporal artery biopsy giant cell arteritis

TAB is considered the gold standard for the diagnosis of GCA, and remains the most specific diagnostic test. It is a low-risk procedure with high diagnostic yield, and therefore a clinical diagnosis should be confirmed by TAB whenever possible, as patients with GCA require long-term glucocorticoid therapy. The classic and most common (80% of positive TABs) histological picture of GCA is characterized by a transmural inflammatory infiltrate consisting of lymphocytes and macrophages (1). Multinucleated giant cells, which are usually located near the internal elastic, are found in 75% of specimens showing transmural infiltration. Plasma cells, eosinophils, and neutrophils are generally inconspicuous (< 10% of TABs with transmural infiltration).

More limited inflammation restricted to the adventitial or periadventitial tissue without medial involvement is generally associated with GCA, and is clinically significant. A retrospective analysis of 317 inflamed TABs from patients with GCA showed that in a significant proportion of biopsies inflammation spared the media and was restricted to the periadventitial small vessels (9%), to the adventitial vasa vasorum (6%), or to the adventitia (6%). Despite lower frequencies of cranial symptoms and halo sign at colour duplex sonography (CDS), and lower levels of acute phase reactants, these more limited patterns of GCA were equally associated with the risk of ischaemic complication as the classic transmural GCA (1, 2).

However, vasculitis in the temporal artery, and particularly in the surrounding periadventitial small vessel, may represent a vasculitis other than GCA. Marked fibrinoid necrosis is not a feature of GCA, and when present it should raise the possibility of a systemic necrotizing vasculitis such as panarteritis nodosa or antineutrophil cytoplasmic antibody-associated vasculitis (1). In the absence of inflammation, other structural changes in the walls of temporal arteries are often present (media–intimal scar, intimal hyperplasia, fragmentation of internal elastic lamina, calcification, adventitial fibrosis, and neoangiogenesis), and some of these have been described as 'healed' or quiescent arteritis (3–5). However, structural, non-inflammatory alterations such as intimal hyperplasia, calcifications, and fragmentation of the internal elastic lamina do not discriminate between patients with GCA and age-matched controls (6, 7). Therefore, the term 'healed arteritis' should be avoided and the definition of a positive TAB be restricted to the biopsies showing inflammation. However, functional changes at TAB may discriminate at least to some extent patients with GCA from those without. In this regard, increased rho kinase activity has been shown to be more prevalent in patients with GCA (regardless of the presence of an inflammatory infiltrate) compared to matched controls (8).

A negative TAB does not rule out GCA, and a diagnosis of biopsy-negative GCA has been reported in 13–44% of patients with clinical GCA, even when TAB is performed accurately (3, 9, 10). There are a number of reasons why TAB may be negative in patients with GCA. Inflammatory changes affect the temporal arteries in a segmental fashion, and skip lesions have been reported in 8.5–28% of TABs from patients with GCA (11, 12). It is likely that such discontinuous inflammatory changes in the temporal artery may cause false-negative biopsy results if the particular vessel segment sampled is not inflamed, especially if the length of the biopsy specimen is too short.

A major issue in reducing the risk of false-negative histological results is the size of the biopsy. The length of the TAB is important in obtaining positive histological findings for GCA. A biopsy specimen longer than 0.7–1 cm significantly increases the diagnostic yield (13, 14). The rate of positive TAB is very low (8%) when TAB length is 5 mm or less, while the rate approaches 50% when TAB length is 11 mm or more, and exceeds 50% with TAB longer than 20 mm (15). Guided by clinical examination, the side with more abnormal findings (headaches and tenderness or nodularity of temporal vessels) should be sampled, since the presence of abnormalities of the temporal artery on physical examination is associated with a high predictive value for a positive TAB (16). In this regard, CDS-guided TAB does not result in a higher frequency of patients with positive TAB compared to a careful physical examination-guided TAB, indicating that CDS is not useful in improving the sensitivity of TAB for the diagnosis of GCA. However, temporal artery CDS may be helpful for marking the segment to be biopsied in cases with small or deeply localized temporal arteries, reducing the risk of missing the artery (17). Since negative unilateral temporal artery biopsy is associated with a very low frequency (1–3%) of a subsequent positive contralateral biopsy, bilateral biopsies are not recommended as a routine procedure (18, 19).

Limited forms of temporal artery inflammation without medial involvement can be subtle, and can be easily missed if particular attention is not paid to the small vessels surrounding the temporal artery. In a retrospective series of inflamed TAB, the first slide was negative (and the lesion was present only in deeper sections) in 50% of peri-adventitial small vessels vasculitis, in 43.5% of adventitial vasa vasorum vasculitis, and in 32% of vasculitis limited to adventitia, but never in classic transmural inflammation (1). For these reasons we suggest obtaining three further slides at different levels if the first slide is negative.

In some patients with GCA the temporal arteries may be truly spared by the inflammatory process. Particularly patients with large-vessel involvement have negative TAB findings in a quite high proportion (42–48%) of cases (20, 21). Finally, glucocorticoids therapy may decrease the rate of positive TAB findings. In newly diagnosed GCA patients treated with high-dose glucocorticoids, TAB was positive in 78% of patients treated for less than 2 weeks, in 65% of those treated for 2–4 weeks, and in 40% of those treated for longer than 4 weeks (22). Therefore, while glucocorticoid therapy should be promptly started if GCA is strongly suspected, it is preferable to perform TAB as soon as possible after onset of glucocorticoid therapy. However, failing to perform TAB within few days after initiation of glucocorticoid therapy should not be a reason to not perform TAB in patients with suspected GCA, since the diagnostic yield of TAB is valuable up to 4 weeks from starting high-dose steroid treatment.

References

1. Cavazza A, Muratore F, Boiardi L, et al. Inflamed temporal artery: histologic findings in 354 biopsies, with clinical correlations. Am J Surg Pathol 2014; 38(10):1360–70.

2. Restuccia G, Cavazza A, Boiardi L, et al. Small-vessel vasculitis surrounding an uninflamed temporal artery and isolated vasa vasorum vasculitis of the temporal artery: two subsets of giant cell arteritis. Arthritis Rheum 2012; 64(2):549–56.

3. Allsop CJ, Gallagher PJ. Temporal artery biopsy in giant-cell arteritis. A reappraisal. Am J Surg Pathol 1981; 5:317–23.

4. Seidman MA, Mitchell RN. Surgical pathology of small- and medium-sized vessels. Surg Pathol 2012; 5:435–51.

5. Lee YC, Padera RF, Noss EH, et al. Clinical course and management of a consecutive series of patients with 'healed temporal arteritis'. J Rheumatol 2012; 39(2):295–302.

6. Cox M, Gilks B. Healed or quiescent temporal arteritis versus senescent changes in temporal artery biopsy specimens. Pathology 2001; 33:163–6.

7. Foss F, Brown L. An elastic Van Gieson stain is unnecessary for the histological diagnosis of giant cell temporal arteritis. J Clin Pathol 2010; 63:1077–9.

8. Lally L, Pernis A, Narula N, et al. Increased rho kinase activity in temporal artery biopsies from patients with giant cell arteritis. Rheumatology 2015; 54:554–8.

9. Roth AM, Milsow L, Keltner JL. The ultimate diagnoses of patients undergoing temporal artery biopsies. Arch Ophthalmol 1984; 102:901–3.

10. Hall S, Persellin S, Lie JT, et al. The therapeutic impact of temporal artery biopsy. Lancet 1983; 2(8361):1217–20.

11. Poller DN, van Wyk Q, Jeffrey MJ. The importance of skip lesions in temporal arteritis. J Clin Pathol 2000; 53:137–9.

12. Klein RG, Campbell RJ, Hunder GG, et al. Skip lesions in temporal arteritis. Mayo Clin Proc 1976; 51:504–10.

13. Ypsilantis E, Courtney ED, Chopra N, et al. Importance of specimen length during temporal artery biopsy. Br J Surg 2011; 98(11):1556–60.

14. Taylor-Gjevre R, Vo M, Shukla D, et al. Temporal artery biopsy for giant cell arteritis. J Rheumatol 2005; 32(7):1279–82.

15. Breuer GS, Nesher R, Nesher G. Effect of biopsy length on the rate of positive temporal artery biopsies. Clin Exp Rheumatol 2009; 27(1 Suppl 52):S10–13.

16. Gonzalez-Gay MA, Garcia-Porrua C, Llorca J, et al. Biopsy-negative giant cell arteritis: clinical spectrum and predictive factors for positive temporal artery biopsy. Semin Arthritis Rheum 2001; 30(4):249–56.

17. Germanò G, Muratore F, Cimino L, et al. Is colour duplex sonography-guided temporal artery biopsy useful in the diagnosis of giant cell arteritis? A randomized study. Rheumatology (Oxford) 2015; 54(3):400–4.

18. Boyev LR, Miller NR, Green WR. Efficacy of unilateral versus bilateral temporal artery biopsies for the diagnosis of giant cell arteritis. Am J Ophthalmol 1999; 128:211–15.

19. Hall JK, Volpe NJ, Galetta SL, et al. The role of unilateral temporal artery biopsy. Ophthalmology 2003; 110:543–8.

20. Brack A, Martinez-Taboada V, Stanson A, *et al.* Disease pattern in cranial and large-vessel giant cell arteritis. *Arthritis Rheum* 1999; 42:311–17.

21. Muratore F, Kermani TA, Crowson CS, *et al.* Large-vessel giant cell arteritis: a cohort study. *Rheumatology (Oxford)* 2015; 54(3):463–70.

22. Narváez J, Bernad B, Roig-Vilaseca D, *et al.* Influence of previous corticosteroid therapy on temporal artery biopsy yield in giant cell arteritis. *Semin Arthritis Rheum* 2007; 37(1):13–19.

Chapter 8

Positron emission tomography and magnetic resonance imaging

Daniel E. Blockmans

Key points

- Fluorine-18-labelled fluorodeoxyglucose-positron emission tomography (FDG-PET) and magnetic resonance imaging (MRI) are two techniques which can be used to diagnose giant cell arteritis when temporal artery biopsy fails to do so.

- Depending on the available equipment and experience, one may choose FDG-PET, MRI, or colour Doppler sonography, especially where the disease does not involve temporal arteries.

- FDG-PET and MRI may strengthen a presumed clinical diagnosis of polymyalgia rheumatica.

8.1 Introduction

PET with the use of 18F-FDG as an isotope enables the visualization of areas of increased glucose metabolism throughout the body. This technique has many applications in oncology, where it is used in the detection and staging of different kind of tumours. As inflammatory lesions also consume more glucose, the diagnostic contribution of FDG-PET in several infectious or inflammatory conditions has also been investigated (1–3). In the late 1990s, it became clear that inflammation of large vessels can be detected by PET (4). The concept of large-vessel giant cell arteritis (GCA) involving principally the larger intrathoracic arteries rather than just the temporal ones evolved around the same time (5). PET scanning has added to our scientific knowledge of GCA and polymyalgia rheumatica (PMR), while earning a place in the clinical practice of doctors caring for patients with GCA and/or PMR.

8.2 What has FDG-PET taught us about giant cell arteritis and polymyalgia rheumatica?

It has been known for decades that GCA can attack other arteries beyond the temporal ones. It was recognized that the aorta can be involved, with the development of thoracic or abdominal aneurysms as a late but potentially lethal consequence (6), or that the subclavian arteries can become stenotic due to GCA, much like in Takayasu's arteritis. It was thought, however, that these were rather rare, atypical complications. With the use of PET, it has been shown that aortic involvement is present in about half of cases, and that the subclavian arteries are more or less inflamed in almost three-quarters of cases (7). Most of these involvements remain asymptomatic but one can assume that, by using even more sensitive methods, large-vessel inflammation in GCA may be noticed in almost every patient. Vascular inflammation in GCA is also seen in the abdominal aorta and the iliac and femoral arteries, even in the arteries below the knee (8). It has also been shown that GCA is a symmetric vasculitis, involving corresponding arteries on both sides of the body and that it occurs simultaneously in different vascular areas (hence, it does not seem to spread starting from one artery) (7). It is known that in most patients, vascular increased FDG uptake subsides after starting steroids, but in some patients, some residual FDG uptake appears to remain (4, 7). It is not certain whether this residual FDG uptake links to residual vasculitic activity, or whether it is caused by 'vascular remodelling', but this topic needs to be explored further. There is indirect evidence from a retrospective study that patients with an increased FDG uptake in the larger thoracic arteries at the time of diagnosis, might be more prone to dilatation of the thoracic aorta several years later, compared to those GCA patients with negative PET scans at diagnosis (9).

In isolated PMR, PET scans showed that patients' complaints are caused by inflammation around the shoulders and hips (explaining shoulder and pelvic stiffness and pain) and by inflammation between the spinous processes of the cervical and lumbar spine (explaining neck and back pain), and not, for example, by inflammation of the axillary arteries (10–12). In about 30% of isolated PMR patients, however, there is some vascular FDG accumulation detectable by PET, especially at the level of the subclavian arteries (10, 11). This illustrates the close relationship between GCA and PMR.

8.3 What is the place of FDG-PET in the diagnosis and management of giant cell arteritis and polymyalgia rheumatica patients in the clinic?

Two case reports in which PET scintigraphy was indispensable are given here as examples for the clinical usefulness of this technique.

A 64-year-old, female patient with a medical history of a hysterectomy, kidney stones, and an operation on the small intestine many years ago, was seen at a general medical consultation because she felt tired and feverish, with a flu-like illness and a dry cough. This was of 7 weeks' duration. Her appetite was low and she had lost 3.5 kg in weight in 5 weeks. There had been an episode of occipital headache 2–3 months ago, but this had cleared completely. Clinical examination was normal, with the exception of a pectus excavatum and a large birthmark. Lung auscultation showed normal vesicular breathing and the liver seemed normal by palpation and percussion. Blood examination showed increased inflammatory parameters (C-reactive protein (CRP) 182 mg/L; erythrocyte sedimentation rate (ESR) 125 mm/h) and slightly disturbed liver function: alanine aminotransferase 39 U/L (normal < 33 U/L), alkaline phosphatases 167 U/L (normal < 103 U/L), and gamma glutamyl transpeptidase 208 U/L (normal < 36 U/L). A FDG-PET scan showed highly increased FDG accumulation at the large blood vessels (Figure 8.1). A temporal artery biopsy (TAB) was normal. The patient was treated with steroids with a quick resolution of all symptoms and normalization of inflammatory parameters and liver function.

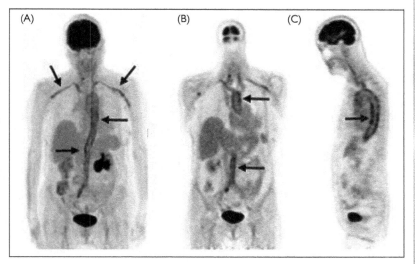

Figure 8.1 The arrows point to the strong FDG uptake in the subclavian arteries (A and B) and in the entire aortic wall (A, B and C), which is visible in the frontal plane (A and B) and in the sagittal plane (C).

A 71-year-old, female patient with a medical history of arterial hypertension, gonarthrosis, hypercholesterolaemia, oesophagitis, and migraine was referred to the general internal medicine department by her general practitioner (GP) for a suspicion of GCA. She had experienced a constant headache for 2.5 months which was clearly different from her known migraine. The GP had noticed a CRP of 34 mg/L and an ESR of 112 mm/hour. A TAB was performed, which was normal. A PET scan showed an increased FDG uptake at the subclavian arteries and in the wall of the thoracic aorta, as well as increased FDG uptake around the shoulders and hips. The headache disappeared quickly after steroids were started.

Due to its limited availability in many countries and the high costs, it is obvious that FDG-PET scintigraphy cannot and should not be performed in most GCA or PMR patients. When patients present with typical symptoms for GCA (headache, visual disturbances, and jaw claudication), GCA is readily suspected and in many cases a temporal biopsy will confirm the presumed diagnosis. However, it is well known that even in 'cranial GCA', temporal biopsy may be negative in up to 25% of patients, due to the segmental nature of the vasculitis (5). Performing a second biopsy on the contralateral side may be another option, but it will only reveal the diagnosis in an additional 3–12% of patients (13). Performing a PET scan may be a valid alternative, or one may prefer to start steroids with only a 'probable diagnosis'. It is the author's experience, however, that these patients with an uncertain diagnosis, in whom steroids were started without biopsy or other proof, frequently relapse while still being on steroids, and problems then start.

In another category of GCA patients, FDG-PET is the first-choice technique to make a diagnosis. GCA can manifest itself very atypically, with only fever, a dry cough, malaise, or weight loss as presenting symptoms. In these patients, GCA is one of several possibilities, which makes FDG-PET scintigraphy indispensable. Although it is an expensive technique, it can make many other examinations superfluous and will shorten the hospital stay considerably when it is performed early.

Of course, a negative PET scan does not exclude the diagnosis of GCA, since in many patients the vasculitis is indeed restricted to the temporal arteries (14). Increased FDG uptake in the temporal arteries cannot be visualized by PET, since these arteries are too small, are too superficially located (there is always an increased signal at the transition between body and air, due to technical reasons), and are too close to the brain, which has a very intense FDG uptake.

In patients with typical PMR symptoms and clearly increased inflammatory parameters, the diagnosis can be made purely on clinical grounds and steroids started. However, symptoms may not be so typical or CRP may be only slightly increased. Finding an increased FDG uptake around the shoulders and hips is compatible with this diagnosis, since it is found in 90% of PMR patients. The diagnosis becomes even more obvious when there is also an increased FDG uptake at the spinous processes of the cervical and/or lumbar spine (Figure 8.2), but these findings are less sensitive since they are found in only 50% of PMR patients (10).

Early-onset rheumatoid arthritis (RA) is an important differential in diagnosing PMR, but PMR can also be a first manifestation of RA. A prospective study on the utility of FDG-PET to differentiate PMR from other diseases is still recruiting patients. Shoulders and neck are frequently involved in both PMR and RA, while more distal synovitis indicates RA. Increased FDG uptake in the larger thoracic vessels is not encountered in RA, but is seen in about 30% of isolated PMR patients (10).

Although PMR is not a paraneoplastic condition, an occult not-related tumour may be found occasionally in these elderly patients by performing a PET scan for the diagnosis of PMR.

There is no need to repeat the FDG-PET scan during the treatment with steroids if symptoms and inflammatory parameters stay away, since results of PET scans will not predict which patients are more prone to relapse. At the time of a possible relapse, a PET scan can be repeated, but vascular and articular FDG uptake frequently is not as intense as at diagnosis, probably due to the effect of previous steroid treatment (7, 10).

8.4 **What are the caveats when interpreting FDG-PET scans for vasculitis?**

Atherosclerosis is also an inflammatory process, and hence it may be visible as an increased FDG uptake in the wall of larger arteries (15, 16). Confusion with vasculitis rarely poses a problem, since atherosclerosis of the aorta can be seen on FDG-PET scintigraphy as localized hot spots, while vasculitis produces a more linear, smooth PET signal. The arteries of the arms are not frequently involved in atherosclerosis, but the differential diagnosis between atherosclerosis and vasculitis may be difficult in the arteries of the legs. Increased FDG uptake in the femoral and more distal arteries is not so specific for vasculitis (Figure 8.3) (17).

Another caveat is that FDG in the blood pool may mimic vasculitis of the subclavian arteries. These arteries are too small to show a clear difference between vascular wall FDG uptake (which equals vasculitis) and FDG still present in the blood flowing through the subclavian arteries. This problem arises when the acquisition time is too low (e.g. 45 minutes) and is much less of a problem when the acquisition time is 90–180 minutes (18). Comparing the intensity of FDG uptake in the different arteries with FDG uptake in the liver (which equals blood flow) and calculating a receiver operating characteristic

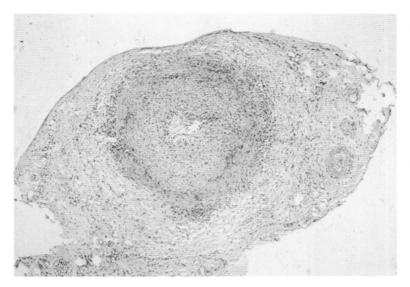

Figure 2.1 (see Figure 2.1 p. 12).

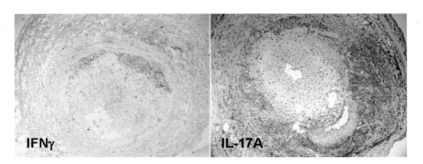

Figure 2.3 (see Figure 2.3 p. 14).

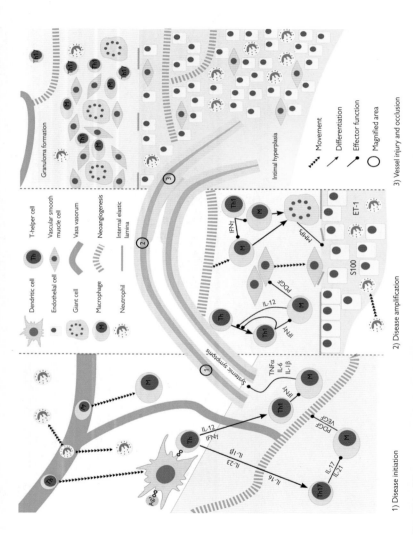

Figure 2.4 (see Figure 2.4 p. 16).

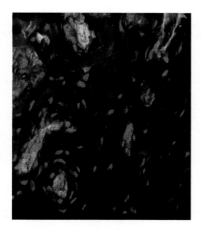

Figure 2.5 (see Figure 2.5 p. 18).

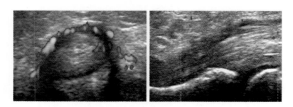

Figure 3.2 (see Figure 3.2 p. 28).

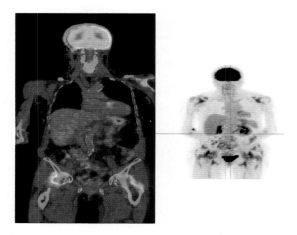

Figure 3.3 (see Figure 3.3 p. 30).

Reproduced from Williams M, Jain S, Patil P, and Dasgupta B, Contribution of imaging in polymyalgia rheumatic, Joint Bone Spine, 2013: 80; 228–9 with permission from Elsevier.

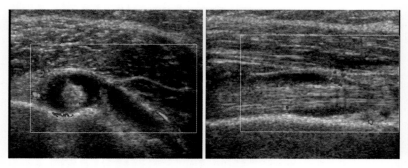

Figure 6.3 (see Figure 6.3 p. 51).

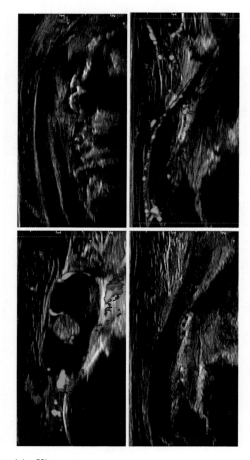

Figure 6.4 (see Figure 6.4 p. 52).

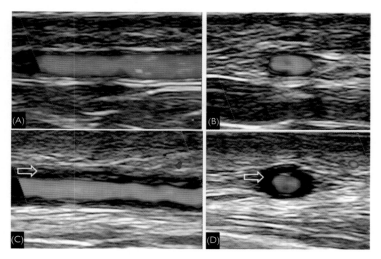

Figure 6.5 (see Figure 6.5 p. 53).

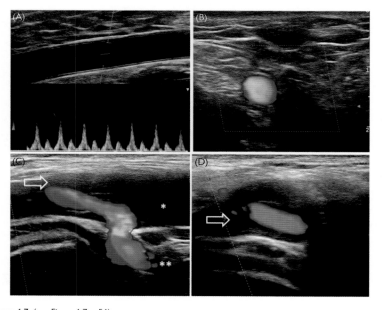

Figure 6.7 (see Figure 6.7 p. 56).

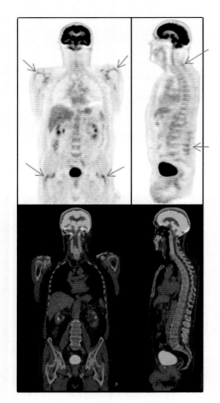

Figure 8.2 (see Figure 8.2 p. 67).

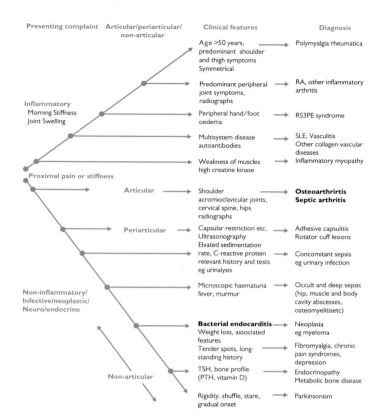

Figure 9.1 (see Figure 9.1 p. 74).

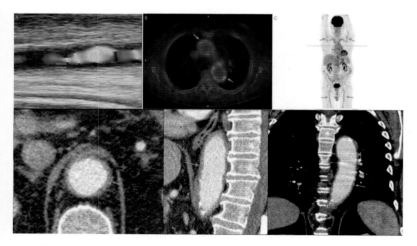

Figure 12.2 (see Figure 12.2 p. 100).

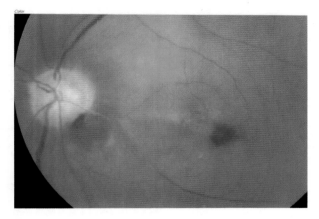

Figure 13.1 (see Figure 13.1 p. 104).

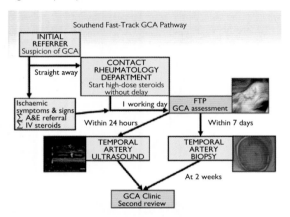

Figure 13.3 (see Figure 13.3 p. 107).

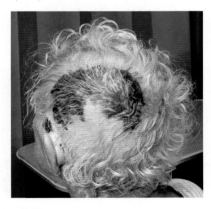

Figure 13.4 (see Figure 13.4 p. 109).

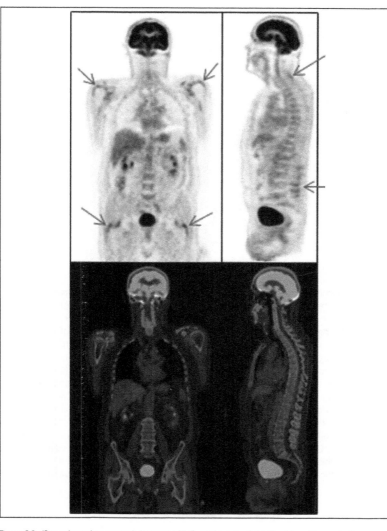

Figure 8.2 (See colour plate section). Increased FDG uptake around the shoulders, hips, and spinous processes of the cervical spine in a patient with isolated PMR (arrows).

analysis-based cut-off ratio might also resolve this issue (19). A cut-off of 1.89 yielded a sensitivity of 80% and a specificity of 79% for GCA diagnosis (20).

FDG-PET scans performed in patients already treated with steroids are hard to interpret, since steroids will dampen FDG uptake in the vascular wall (7, 21). Therefore, it is important to start steroid treatment only after performing the PET scan, if one wants

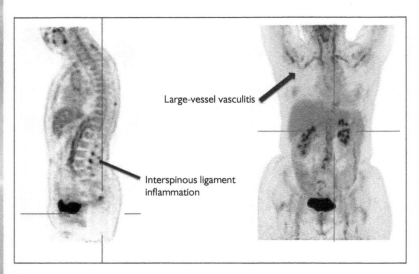

Large-vessel vasculitis

Interspinous ligament
inflammation

Figure 8.3 FDG-PET scan in a patient with PMR with large-vessel vasculitis.

to do this examination. Thus, in patients with visual symptoms (amaurosis fugax) in whom steroid treatment is urgent, there is no time to perform a PET scan.

In patients with diabetes, blood sugar levels before the injection of FDG ideally should be under 140 mg/dL, which can be achieved if necessary with the aid of intravenous insulin. If blood sugar levels are too high (especially if higher than 200 mg/dL), interpretation of images becomes problematic due to competition of FDG and glucose.

The most recent machines combine PET with computed tomography (CT) scanning. For the diagnosis of GCA or PMR, the CT modality is not in fact needed. However, aortic wall thickening can be detected as a possible complication of GCA at diagnosis or aortic dilatation at follow-up (22). Always ask that the patient remains with their arms alongside their body, since this allows the best interpretation of FDG accumulation in the axillary arteries and around the shoulder (frequently, on performing a combined PET/CT scan, the patient is asked to elevate their arms in order to lower radiation, but this position makes PET interpretation more difficult). In the near future, machines in which PET and MRI modalities are combined will become available.

8.5 What can magnetic resonance add to the diagnosis or assessment of giant cell arteritis and polymyalgia rheumatica?

Magnetic resonance angiography (MRA) with gadolinium nowadays almost completely replaces the formerly used classical angiography, which was invasive and needed rather large amounts of possibly toxic contrast products. MRA can demonstrate the typically long, smooth stenosis or occlusions of the distal subclavian and axillary arteries (Figure 8.4A). Aortic involvement, both at diagnosis with aortic wall thickening (Figure 8.4B) and during follow-up with possible aneurysm formation, can also be detected by MRI. High signal intensity in the aortic wall detected by a post-gadolinium, T1-weighted image sequence indicates acute inflammatory tissue damage, both in Takayasu's arteritis

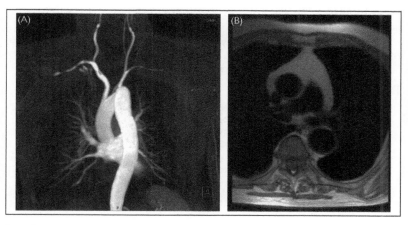

Figure 8.4 (A) Magnetic resonance angiography in a 74-year-old patient with GCA and severe claudication in both arms showing stenoses and occlusions of both subclavian arteries. (B) MRI of the same patient showing a thickened wall of the descending thoracic aorta.

(23) and in GCA (24). Magnetic resonance is not a first-line technique to diagnose GCA, but once the diagnosis is made by other means (biopsy, temporal artery ultrasound examination, or FDG-PET), magnetic resonance may be used to show vascular involvement in different areas in greater detail. While the temporal arteries themselves cannot be visualized by FDG-PET due to technical reasons, MRI appeared to be well suitable for visualizing vessel wall inflammation in the temporal arteries or the superficial occipital arteries. Diagnostic criteria for inflamed vessel wall segments are thickening of the wall and increased mural gadolinium-based contrast enhancement. The intensity of this inflammatory hyper-enhancement decreases significantly under corticosteroid therapy (25). High-resolution MRI can even detect mural inflammation of intradural branches of the internal carotid arteries (26), which are only exceptionally involved in GCA (27). Bley et al. reported a sensitivity of 80.6% and specificity of 97.0% for contrast-enhanced high-resolution MRI of the temporal and occipital arteries for the diagnosis of GCA, as compared to clinical diagnosis (28), which could make a TAB unnecessary if this MRI technique is readily available.

In PMR, MRI can show bursal and joint synovitis, associated or not with tenosynovitis. Bilateral subdeltoid/subacromial bursitis, glenohumeral synovitis, biceps tenosynovitis, and trochanteric bursitis occur more in PMR than in control patients (29). MRI studies confirmed that bursitis of interspinous joints of the cervical spine causes the neck pain in PMR (30). A moderate to marked (grade 2 or more on a semiquantitative 0–3 scale) cervical bursitis occurred significantly more frequently in 13 patients with PMR than in 12 control patients with other causes of neck pain (fibromyalgia, cervical osteoarthritis, or spondyloarthritis) (83.3% compared with 30.7%, P = 0.015).

8.6 Conclusion

FDG-PET and MRI are two techniques which can be used to diagnose GCA when TAB fails to do so. Depending on the available equipment and experience, one may choose FDG-PET, MRI, or colour Doppler sonography, which is described elsewhere (see Chapter 6). Since GCA does not always involve the temporal arteries, TAB has lost its status of being a gold standard for the diagnosis of this form of vasculitis.

FDG-PET and MRI—like echography—may strengthen a presumed clinical diagnosis of PMR.

References

1. Brudin LH, Valind SO, Rhodes CG, et al. Fluorine-18 deoxyglucose uptake in sarcoidosis measured with positron emission tomography. Eur J Nucl Med 1994; 21:297–305.

2. Ichiya Y, Kuwabara Y, Sasaki M, et al. FDG-PET in infectious lesions: the detection and assessment of lesion activity. Ann Nucl Med 1996; 10:185–91.

3. Blockmans D, Knockaert D, Maes A, et al. Clinical value of (18)fluoro-deoxyglucose positron emission tomography for patients with fever of unknown origin. Clin Infect Dis 2001; 32:191–6.

4. Blockmans D, Maes A, Stroobants S, et al. New arguments for a vasculitic nature of polymyalgia rheumatic using positron emission tomography. Rheumatology 1999; 38:444–7.

5. Brack A, Martinez-Taboada V, Stanson A, et al. Disease pattern in cranial and large-vessel giant cell arteritis. Arthritis Rheum 1999; 42:311–17.

6. Evans JM, O'Fallon WM, Hunder GG. Increased incidence of aortic aneurysm and dissection in giant cell (temporal) arteritis. A population based study. Ann Intern Med 1995; 122:502–7.

7. Blockmans D, De Ceuninck L, Vanderschueren S, et al. Repetitive 18F-fluorodeoxyglucose positron emission tomography in giant cell arteritis: a prospective study of 35 patients. Arthritis Rheum 2006; 55:131–7.

8. Tato F, Hoffmann U. Clinical presentation and vascular imaging in giant cell arteritis of the femoropopliteal and tibioperoneal arteries. Analysis of four cases. J Vasc Surg 2006; 44:176–82.

9. Blockmans D, Coudyzer W, Vanderschueren S, et al. Relationship between fluorodeoxyglucose uptake in the large vessels and late aortic diameter in giant cell arteritis. Rheumatology 2008; 47:1179–84.

10. Blockmans D, De Ceuninck L, Vanderschueren S, et al. Repetitive 18-fluorodeoxyflucose positron emission tomography in isolated polymyalgia rheumatica: a prospective study in 35 patients. Rheumatology 2007; 46:672–7.

11. Yamashita H, Kubota K, Takahashi Y, et al. Whole-body fluoro-deoxyglucose positron emission tomography/computed tomography in patients with active polymyalgia rheumatica: evidence for distinctive bursitis and large-vessel vasculitis. Mod Rheumatol 2012; 22:705–11.

12. Adams H, Raijmakers P, Smulders Y. Polymyalgia rheumatica and interspinous FDG uptake on PET/CT. Clin Nucl Med 2012; 37:502–5.

13. Breuer GS, Nesher G, Nesher R. Rate of discordant findings in bilateral temporal artery biopsy to diagnose giant cell arteritis. J Rheumatol 2009; 36:794–6.

14. Brodmann M, Lipp R, Passath A, et al. The role of 2-18F-fluoro-2-deoxy-D-glucose positron emission tomography in the diagnosis of giant cell arteritis of the temporal arteries. Rheumatology 2004; 43:241–2.

15. Yun M, Jang S, Cucchiara A, et al. 18F FDG uptake in the large arteries: a correlation study with the atherogenic risk factors. Semin Nucl Med 2002; 32:70–6.

16. Kang S, Kyung C, Park JS, et al. Subclinical vascular inflammation in subjects with normal weight obesity and its association with body fat: an 18F-FDG-PET/CT study. Cardiovasc Diabetol 2014; 13:70–81.

17. Blockmans D, Stroobants S, Maes A, et al. Positron emission tomography in giant cell arteritis and polymyalgia rheumatica: evidence for inflammation of the aortic arch. Am J Med 2000; 108:246–9.

18. Martinez-Rodriguez I, Del Castillo-Matos R, Quirce R, *et al*. Aortic 18F-FDG PET/CT uptake pattern at 60 min (early) and 180 min (delayed) acquisition in a control population: a visual and semiquantitative comparative analysis. *Nucl Med Comm* 2013; 34:926–30.

19. Hautzel H, Sander O, Heinzel A, *et al*. Assessment of large-vessel involvement in giant cell arteritis with 18F-FDG PET; introducing a ROC-analysis-based cut-off ratio. *J Nucl Med* 2008; 49:1107–13.

20. Prieto-Gonzalez S, Depetris M, Garcia-Martinez A, *et al*. Positron emission tomography assessment of large vessel inflammation in patients with newly diagnosed, biopsy-proven giant cell arteritis: a prospective, case-control study. *Ann Rheum Dis* 2014; 73:1388–92.

21. Both M, Ahmadi-Simab K, Reuter M, *et al*. MRI and FDG-PET in the assessment of inflammatory aortic arch syndrome in complicated courses of giant cell arteritis. *Ann Rheum Dis* 2008; 67:1030–3.

22. Prieto-Gonzalez S, Arguis P, Garcia-Martinez A, *et al*. Large vessel involvement in biopsy-proven giant cell arteritis: prospective study in 40 newly diagnosed patients using CT angiography. *Ann Rheum Dis* 2012; 71:1170–6.

23. Desai MY, Stone JH, Foo TK, *et al*. Delayed contrast enhanced MRI of the aortic wall in Takayasu's arteritis: initial experience. *AJR Am J Roentgenol* 2005; 184:1427–31.

24. Sabater EA, Stanson AW. Cross-sectional imaging in vasculitis. In Baal GV, Fessler BJ, Bridges SL Jr (eds) *Oxford Textbook of Vasculitis* (3rd ed). Oxford: Oxford University Press, 2014:247–65.

25. Blockmans D, Bley T, Schmidt W. Imaging for large-vessel vasculitis. *Curr Opin Rheumatol* 2009; 21:19–28.

26. Siemonsen C, Brekenfeld C, Holst B, *et al*. 3T MRI reveals extra- and intracranial involvement in giant cell arteritis. *AJNR Am J Neuroradiol* 2015; 36(1):91–7.

27. Salvarani C, Giannini C, Miller DV, *et al*. Giant cell arteritis: involvement of intracranial arteries. *Arthritis Rheum* 2006; 55:985–9.

28. Bley TA, Uhl M, Carew J, *et al*. Diagnostic value of high-resolution MR imaging in giant cell arteritis. *AJNR Am J Neuroradiol* 2007; 28:1722–7.

29. Camellino D, Cimmino MA. Imaging of polymyalgia rheumatica: indications on its pathogenesis, diagnosis and prognosis. *Rheumatology* 2012; 51:77–86.

30. Salvarani C, Barozzi L, Cantini F, *et al*. Cervical interspinous bursitis in active polymyalgia rheumatica. *Ann Rheum Dis* 2008; 67:758–61.

Chapter 9

Differential diagnosis

Dario Camellino and Marco A. Cimmino

Key points

- The main differential diagnosis of polymyalgia rheumatica is elderly-onset rheumatoid arthritis, followed by calcium pyrophosphate deposition disease and infections.
- Giant cell arteritis should be differentiated from other, less frequent vasculitides and from neurological diseases.
- History taking, clinical examination, laboratory tests, and imaging help in differential diagnosis.

9.1 Differential diagnosis of polymyalgia rheumatica

Polymyalgia rheumatica (PMR) is an inflammatory disease of the elderly characterized by the non-specific findings of girdle pain and stiffness and constitutional symptoms: as a result its differential diagnosis ranges from rheumatic to infective and neoplastic diseases (Figure 9.1). PMR and giant cell arteritis (GCA) account for about 8–12% of cases of fever of unknown origin. PMR patients often undergo many examinations before a correct diagnosis is established and about one-third of them experience hospitalization. They also often show peripheral arthritis, which further complicates the diagnosis. In a cohort of 61 patients with polymyalgic features, a diagnostic shift was observed in 32 (52%): calcium pyrophosphate deposition disease (CPPD) was diagnosed in nine patients, elderly-onset rheumatoid arthritis (EORA) in 18, and elderly-onset spondyloarthritis in five. Ultrasonographic clues for the diagnosis of PMR were the presence of subacromial-subdeltoid bursitis, low frequency of knee menisci chondrocalcinosis, and low Power-Doppler scores at the wrist. Conversely, effusion and synovitis of wrist, metacarpophalangeal joints, metatarsophalangeal joints, and tendinous calcaneal calcifications or Achilles enthesitis were more frequent in patients with diagnoses other than PMR.

9.1.1 Differential diagnosis with other rheumatic diseases

9.1.1.1 Elderly-onset rheumatoid arthritis

The main differential diagnosis in patients with suspected PMR is EORA, which also may present with girdle pain and raised inflammation. Both conditions also share a common genetic background and patients with cured PMR can relapse as EORA. Many

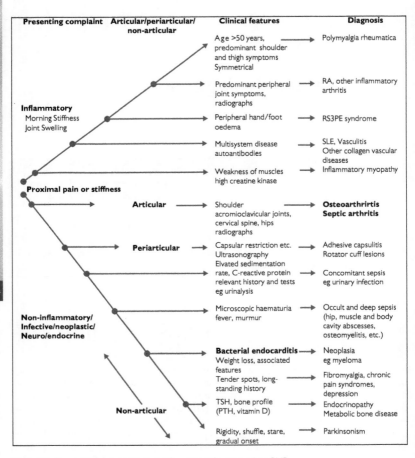

Figure 9.1 (See colour plate section). A safe and specific approach to PMR.

studies have addressed clinical and laboratory discriminating clues, with only peripheral arthritis being effective. However, peripheral arthritis, being present in up to 40% of PMR patients, has a poor predictive value. In addition, immunoglobulin M rheumatoid factor is not rare in healthy elderly subject, preceding the onset of PMR. Conversely, the finding of anticyclic citrullinated peptide antibodies is strongly related to EORA. In a study with fluorine-18-labelled fluorodeoxyglucose-positron emission tomography/ computed tomography (FDG-PET/CT), PMR patients showed higher uptake of the ischiatic, trochanteric, and interspinous bursae compared to EORA patients. Shoulders were not evaluated because of their anatomical complexity and the difficulty of precisely localizing inflammation. In the clinic, follow-up over time is often the only way to help differential diagnosis: if glucocorticoid treatment is effective despite its tapering and peripheral arthritis does not become chronic, the diagnosis of PMR is likely to be correct.

9.1.1.2 *Seronegative spondyloarthritides*

Elderly-onset spondyloarthropathies can sometimes present with pronounced morning stiffness and girdle involvement. If these patients are misdiagnosed as PMR, the lack of response to glucocorticoids may suggest the correct diagnosis. In addition, the tests commonly used for spondyloarthropathies, such as human leucocyte antigen B27 and magnetic resonance imaging of the spine and sacroiliac joints, can help. A more subtle link between these conditions may exist, as suggested by old imaging studies, showing involvement of the sternoclavicular and sacroiliac joints in patients with PMR.

9.1.1.3 *Remitting seronegative symmetrical synovitis with pitting oedema*

Remitting seronegative symmetrical synovitis with pitting oedema (RS3PE) is a distinct form of arthritis, which primarily affects elderly men. It is characterized by symmetrical distal synovitis, pitting oedema of the dorsum of the hands and/or feet, absence of rheumatoid factor, and an excellent response to glucocorticoids. It has been described in association with many rheumatic conditions, including rheumatoid arthritis and psoriatic arthritis, but the most frequent association is with PMR and EORA. A link between RS3PE and cancer has been also suggested, but not confirmed. In a retrospective studies on 28 RS3PE patients and 123 PMR patients, no differences were found in terms of disease course and treatment response. RS3PE patients were more frequently males and smokers.

9.1.1.4 *Microcrystalline arthritis*

Both PMR and CPPD are diseases of old age. If proximal joints are involved in CPPD, symptoms can resemble those of PMR. In a cohort of 118 patients with 'PMR presenting features', 36 met criteria for both PMR and CPPD and the best predictors for the presence of CPPD were age at diagnosis, tibiofemoral osteoarthritis, tendon calcifications, and ankle arthritis. Unfortunately, only 12 of the patients diagnosed as CPPD underwent synovial fluid analysis. Crowned dens syndrome, a condition defined by the association of periodic acute cervico-occipital pain with fever, neck stiffness, raised inflammatory markers, and calcifications of the cruciform ligament around the odontoid process, may mimic PMR, GCA, or meningitis. Diagnosis is established by careful history taking, as CPPD is frequently intermittent, and by the observation of the calcification by CT. In the polymyalgic patient with synovial fluid effusion, its analysis is important in view of the high prevalence of CPPD.

9.1.1.5 *Polymyositis*

Both PMR and polymyositis (PM) involve girdles and proximal muscles: the principal clue for differential diagnosis is the predominance of pain over weakness for PMR and the opposite for PM. Nevertheless, it is not always easy to differentiate stiffness, weakness, and functional impairment. Serum creatine phosphokinase, which is elevated in almost all PM patients, is normal in PMR.

9.1.1.6 *Vasculitides*

GCA is the most frequent form of systemic vasculitis sharing with PMR genetic, demographic, geographic, and ethnic characteristics. Among the remaining vasculitides, small-vessel vasculitides, and in particular microscopic polyangiitis (MPA), may sometimes show similarities with PMR. In a cohort of 86 patients with small-vessel vasculitis, 11 (13%) had a prior diagnosis of PMR. Poor response to glucocorticoid therapy and the presence of mild renal impairment may suggest MPA, although this latter finding is frequent in the age range of PMR. If diagnostic doubts persist, urinalysis for haematuria and proteinuria, and antineutrophil cytoplasmic antibody testing, which is positive in up to 90% of MPA patients, can help.

9.1.2 **Differential diagnosis with other diseases**

9.1.2.1 *Infections*

In patients presenting with polyarthralgia, malaise, and fever, infections must be ruled out promptly. In our experience, bacterial endocarditis is frequently misdiagnosed as PMR. A history of preceding invasive manoeuvres and a cardiac murmur are hints to the correct diagnosis. Serum procalcitonin is usually high in infectious diseases, but was normal in a cohort of 46 patients with PMR and GCA.

9.1.2.2 *Cancer*

The existence of a paraneoplastic form of PMR is debated, with contrasting results in different studies. Several case reports regard the 'PMR-like' presentation of renal cell carcinoma. Clues to the correct diagnosis are the often atypical clinical features of these patients, such as absence of morning stiffness, of limitation of shoulder motion, of typical findings at ultrasonography, and lack of response to glucocorticoids.

A link between PMR and haematological malignancies before, during, or after PMR has been suggested in one study and considered unlikely in another. The standardized incidence ratio of Hodgkin lymphoma after PMR was 2.2 (95% confidence interval 1.4–3.5) and that for non-Hodgkin lymphoma was 1.4 (95% confidence interval 1.2–1.6). A recent cohort study in the United Kingdom showed that PMR patients were significantly more likely than controls to develop cancer with a 69% increased risk, but only during the first 6 months after diagnosis. This finding probably suggests that PMR-like systemic features in patients with cancer can lead to misdiagnosis.

9.1.2.3 *Thyroid disease*

Hypothyroidism may be a possible cause of myalgia and malaise. In a prospective study of 287 patients with PMR and GCA, determination of thyroid hormones was performed in 142 patients. Five of them (3.5%) had hypothyroidism, already diagnosed in three. In a study on 69 PMR and eight GCA patients, none showed biochemical evidence of hypothyroidism and one had clear hyperthyroidism.

9.2 **Differential diagnosis of giant cell arteritis**

GCA is the most frequent type of systemic vasculitis. Its presentations range from inflammatory systemic syndromes (malaise, fever, loss of weight) to ischaemic events, often revealed by headache and visual disturbances. Inflammatory markers are useful in supporting the diagnosis of GCA, presenting high sensitivity (84% for an elevated erythrocyte sedimentation rate and 86% for an elevated C-reactive protein), but lacking specificity (about 30%). GCA at onset can present as fever of unknown origin, a setting where blood cultures are recommended to exclude infection.

FDG-PET has shown a high prevalence of large-vessel vasculitis in GCA patients, but has also revealed the existence of a subgroup of patients characterized by isolated uptake in the thoracic aorta in the absence of other GCA features. In a small cohort of 11 patients with 'isolated aortitis', a predominant male involvement was seen, age at diagnosis was lower, and systemic symptoms were frequent.

9.2.1 Differential diagnosis of acute visual disturbance

The most common ocular manifestation of GCA is visual loss, followed by diplopia, ptosis, and ophthalmoplegia. The underlying mechanisms include mainly anterior ischaemic optic neuropathy, but also occlusion of the central retinal and cilioretinal arteries, ocular ischaemic, and infarction syndromes, and posterior ischaemic optic neuropathy may occur.

Visual field loss is typically sudden and painless. It can be classified on the basis of its duration, the monocular or binocular involvement, and associated symptoms. It is conventionally divided into transient or persistent. In the first case, also known as amaurosis fugax, it is often difficult to identify the underlying cause. This may be embolic (atherosclerosis, dissections, etc.), haemodynamic (malignant hypertension, primary or secondary hypotension, papilloedema, vasospasm), or due to central nervous system involvement (migraine, vertebrobasilar ischaemia, epilepsy). In contrast to GCA, the incidence of transient monocular visual loss in patients aged 50 years or more is higher among males. Transient visual disturbance lasting few seconds is typical of papilloedema whereas other causes induce a visual loss lasting from 2 to 60 minutes, with a mean of 1–15 minutes for thromboembolic events and 10–30 minutes for migraine. The duration of GCA visual disturbances varies, being a few seconds in some cases and permanent in others. Visual disturbance in GCA is typically monocular but, if blindness occurs and is left untreated, it will become bilateral in 25–50% of patients, with a time interval of 1–14 days. Transient visual loss can be described by the patient as blurring, fogging, or as complete darkness: the latter is most frequent in GCA, involving only a part or the entire visual field. Photopsias or scintillations, which can be seen also with closed eyes, suggest a central nervous system origin, such as migraine, or seizures affecting the visual cortex. No single feature is completely typical of GCA. The presence of associated jaw claudication, polymyalgia, and elevation of inflammatory markers make the diagnosis of GCA likely.

The second category of acute visual loss is persistent for more than 24 hours. This condition can originate in the media (keratitis, corneal oedema, hyphaema, lens changes, vitreous haemorrhage, uveitis), retina (retinal artery or vein occlusion, retinal detachment, acute maculopathy), optic nerve (ischaemic optic neuropathy, optic neuritis), and brain (cortical blindness). The presence of pain suggests keratitis, acute glaucoma, or optic neuritis. The presence of redness is typical of keratitis, acute glaucoma, and uveitis. GCA can present with central artery occlusion or with ischaemic optic neuropathy. About 7–18% of patients with anterior ischaemic optic neuropathy present with amaurosis fugax prior to persistent visual loss.

9.2.2 Differential diagnosis of headache

Headache is present in at least two-thirds of GCA patients. GCA should be considered in the differential diagnosis of any new-onset headache occurring in individuals over the age of 50 years. The typical localization is temporal, but occipital, parietal, and frontal areas can also be involved, as well as the whole scalp. Its course can be worsening or fluctuating.

The differential diagnosis of headache is complex because of the high frequency in the general population and its association with many conditions. If neurological signs are present, subarachnoid haemorrhage must be suspected. However, up to 20% of patients presenting at the emergency department with headache and normal neurological examination have subarachnoid haemorrhage. Headache in this setting has a typically acute onset, is generally localized in the nuchal region or behind the orbits, and is described as unusual, and of very high intensity. Fever is a common feature of GCA, but even more common in meningitis. Malaise and weight loss may suggest GCA, but also metastatic cancer with cranial localization. Vomiting is associated with migraine, subarachnoid haemorrhage, and brain tumours, but is uncommon in GCA. Migraine of new onset is uncommon in old patients. Migraine attacks are stereotyped, with pulsating pain present in a well-defined area. Tensive headache is generally described as 'a circle around the head' and lasts days or weeks with a gravative, constrictive pain.

9.2.3 Differential diagnosis with other vasculitides

Takayasu's arteritis (TAK) and GCA are large-vessel vasculitides sharing a predilection for females and the same pathological changes. The distinction between them is mainly based on age, which is less than 50 years in TAK. In a retrospective review of 75 patients with TAK and 69 with GCA, the frequency of fever and arthralgia was similar, but myalgia was more frequent in GCA. Also headache, jaw claudication, and visual blurring were more frequent in GCA, but not exclusive of it, being present in 52%, 5%, and 8% of TAK patients, respectively. Blindness was present only in GCA patients, whereas upper extremity claudication and pulselessness were more frequent in TAK. A recent angiographic study showed a similar arterial involvement, except for carotid and mesenteric arteries, more frequently affected in TAK, and axillary arteries, more frequently affected in GCA.

Temporal arteritis, sometimes used as a synonym of GCA, can occur in other vasculitides, such as granulomatosis with polyangiitis (GPA, formerly Wegener's granulomatosis), polyarteritis nodosa, and other necrotizing vasculitides. Pathological lesions of the temporal artery typical of GCA are absent, at least in GPA. Clues to a correct diagnosis are the concomitant presence of pulmonary and renal involvement, and antineutrophil cytoplasmic antibody positivity.

Further readings

Camellino D, Cimmino MA. Imaging of polymyalgia rheumatica: indications on its pathogenesis, diagnosis and prognosis. *Rheumatology (Oxford)* 2012; 51:77–86.

Dasgupta B, Cimmino MA, Maradit-Kremers H, *et al.* 2012 provisional classification criteria for polymyalgia rheumatica: a European League Against Rheumatism/American College of Rheumatology collaborative initiative. *Ann Rheum Dis* 2012; 71:484–92.

Weyand C, Goronzy J. Giant-cell arteritis and polymyalgia rheumatica. *N Engl J Med* 2014; 371:50–7.

Part 3

Guidelines for treatment

10 Glucocorticoids	81
11 Role of steroid-sparing agents	89
12 Treatment of a relapse and approach to difficult-to-treat patients	97
13 Management of sight loss and other disease- and treatment-related complications	103

Chapter 10

Glucocorticoids

Frank Buttgereit

> **Key points**
>
> - Both the *genomic* and *non-genomic* effects of glucocorticoids (GCs) contribute to successful treatment of polymyalgia rheumatica (PMR) and giant cell arteritis (GCA).
> - Initial treatment for PMR is the minimum effective GC dose within a range of 12.5–25 mg prednisone equivalent daily; for GCA, 40–60 mg/day prednisone equivalent (in case of pending ischaemic complications, intravenous pulse therapy with 500–1000 mg methylprednisolone for 3 days) is initially recommended.
> - A usual treatment course lasts upwards of 1–2 years in both diseases.

10.1 Mechanisms of glucocorticoid actions

GCs form the mainstay of therapy for PMR and GCA since they exert strong anti-inflammatory and immunosuppressive effects. In order to understand their established effectiveness in these (and many other) diseases, a short description of their underlying mechanisms of action may be helpful. This seems to be especially appropriate in this context since very different dosages are used in the treatment of PMR and GCA, ranging from pulse therapy with grams of methylprednisolone (MP) in complicated GCA to maintenance treatment in PMR with very low dosages of 5 mg/day or less prednisone equivalent.

GCs exert their main anti-inflammatory and immunosuppressive effects primarily on leucocytes, where their function as well as their distribution is affected (1). These anti-inflammatory and immunosuppressive effects are primarily produced via so called *genomic* mechanisms, that is, the classical mechanism of action mediated by the cytosolic glucocorticoid receptor (cGCR) (Figure 10.1) (2).

The higher the administered GC dose, the more cGCRs are recruited, and the more intense are the effects induced. This genomic mechanism of GC action can be divided into the *transactivation* and the *transrepression* processes. The so-called transrepression results in a *decreased* expression of pro-inflammatory cytokines while the *increased* synthesis of anti-inflammatory (and other) proteins is termed 'transactivation' (3–6) (Figure 10.1; further details on molecular mechanisms of GC action are described in our recent review (7)).

Some clinical GC effects—especially after intravenous or intra-articular injection of high GC doses—occur too fast to be triggered by the genomic mechanism (4, 8–13).

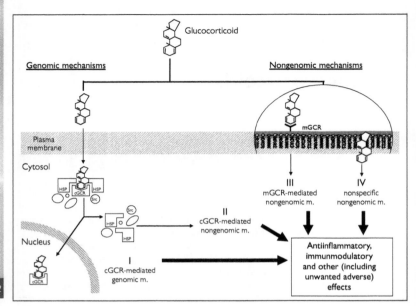

Figure 10.1 Genomic and non-genomic glucocorticoid mechanisms of action.
Reproduced from Buttgereit F, Straub RH, Wehling M, Burmester GR. Glucocorticoids in the treatment of rheumatic diseases: an update on the mechanisms of action. *Arthritis and Rheumatism*. 2004;50(11):3408–3417 with permission from John Wiley and Sons.

This can be explained by the fact that GCs can also mediate rapidly occurring *non-genomic* actions which are mediated via (a) non-specific interactions of GCs with cellular membranes, (b) non-genomic effects mediated by the cGCR, and (c) specific interactions with a membrane-bound glucocorticoid receptor (mGCR; Figure 10.1). Moreover, it should be noted that saturation of all cGCRs is almost complete with 100 mg prednisone equivalent a day, so that specificity, that is, the exclusivity of receptor-mediated effects, is lost at high clinically relevant GC concentrations.

These considerations are important to understand why in GCA, GCs are used at very high concentrations in case of pending ischaemic complications. With intravenous pulse therapy (e.g. 500–1000 mg MP for 3 days), the high GC concentrations achieved are able to mediate clinically relevant non-genomic effects which *rapidly and in addition to* the genomic effects contribute to the clinical success. For example, the above-mentioned, non-specific, non-genomic actions occur in the form of physicochemical interactions with biological membranes. In greater detail, this means that at these very high concentrations there is a non-specific intercalation of GC molecules into cell membranes, altering cell functions by influencing cation transport through the plasma membrane and by increasing the proton leak of the mitochondria. The resulting inhibition of calcium and sodium cycling across the plasma membrane of immune cells is thought to contribute to rapid immunosuppression and to a reduction in the activity of inflammatory processes (2, 7). For this reason, the domains of high-dose GC therapy are ischaemic complications in GCA, but—with the same arguments—also acute exacerbations of life-threatening diseases and therapeutically resistant clinical conditions of varying aetiology.

From these considerations, there are a couple of take-home messages relevant for the treatment of PMR and GCA with GCs:

1. Therapeutically most important for the therapy for PMR and GCA are the classical *genomic* mechanisms which are mediated via the cGCR. These effects occur at any dosages, also at very low ones; but the higher the dosage, the more receptors are activated and the stronger are the GC effects.

2. At higher GC dosages (as with pulse therapy in GCA), rapid non-genomic effects also come into play which contribute to the therapeutic success.

10.2 **Glucocorticoid treatment**

While the effectiveness of GCs in the treatment of PMR and GCA is well established, there are different views on what is the best therapeutic regimen. Daily dosing is preferable to alternate dosing, but there are the following practical questions to which different answers currently exist:

10.2.1 **What initial dose and which tapering regimen are most optimal?**

There is a common understanding that for treatment of PMR, a low GC starting dose should be preferred and that subsequent tapering should be gradual.

Recently published European League Against Rheumatism/American College of Rheumatology (EULAR/ACR) recommendations suggest the minimum effective dose within a range of 12.5–25 mg/day prednisolone (14). A higher initial prednisone dose within this range may be considered in patients with a high risk of relapse (e.g. patients with high erythrocyte sedimentation rate and/or peripheral arthritis) and low risk of adverse events, whereas in patients with relevant comorbidities (e.g. diabetes, osteoporosis, and glaucoma) and other risk factors for GC-related side effects (e.g. female sex), a lower dose may be preferred. Given that a response to this initial therapy is achieved, the dose should be tapered gradually reaching 10 mg/day prednisone equivalent within 4–8 weeks; thereafter (assuming remission of the disease), the daily dose should be decreased by 1 mg every 4 weeks or similar until discontinuation.

The national guidelines by the British Society for Rheumatology (BSR) propose an initial dose of 15 mg/day prednisone equivalent per day for 3 weeks, then taper by 12.5 mg/day (3 weeks) to 10 mg/day (4–6 weeks), and then reduce the daily dose by 1 mg every 4–8 weeks (15). Dutch guidelines also recommend 15 mg/day as an initial dose and then slow tapering at an unspecified rate. In contrast, in Germany, the initial recommended dose is 25 mg/day, followed by a reduction of the daily dose by 2.5 mg per week, and then slowing the taper by reducing the daily dose by 1 mg each month (16).

All these recommendations are not directly supported by evidence because only a single open randomized controlled trial (RCT) on 39 PMR patients compared starting doses of 20 mg/day prednisolone and 10 mg/day prednisolone (17). In the higher-dose group, a lower relapse rate was found at 2 months whereas the effect of different initial GC doses on long-term outcomes is unknown. From retrospective studies, we have limited evidence suggesting a higher risk of adverse events in patients receiving initial GC doses above 15 mg/day prednisone compared to those treated with a lower dose (5, 6).

Different tapering regimens have not been compared in clinical studies so far. A retrospective study suggested that rapid GC tapering (as determined by a 'tapering constant' in regression analysis) was linked with a higher risk of relapse than slower tapering (18). It should be noted that intramuscular MP given every 3 weeks is considered an effective alternate treatment strategy and can be used (e.g. in patients where a lower cumulative GC dose is desirable) (19, 20).

For GCA, EULAR recommends initial treatment with 1 mg/kg/day oral prednisone equivalent; however, a dose of 60 mg/day is usually not exceeded. Similarly, BSR guidelines suggest a starting dose of 40–60 mg/day. GC 'pulse' therapy with intravenous MP 500–1000 mg daily for 3–5 days is considered in patients with pending visual loss or amaurosis fugax (BSR guidelines). In case of amaurosis of one eye, high-dose oral prednisolone (60 mg/day) should be prescribed to protect the contralateral eye.

As in PMR, there is a consensus about a gradual tapering of GCs in GCA. EULAR recommends a target dose of 10–15 mg/day prednisone equivalent after 3 months explicitly discouraging tapering in the form of alternate-day treatment because of a higher relapse risk. BSR recommends to keep the initial dose for 3–4 weeks, then to reduce by 10 mg every 2 weeks to 20 mg, thereafter by 2.5 mg every 2–4 weeks to 10 weeks, and then by 1 mg every 1–2 months assuming that patients are in remission.

As in PMR, there are no solid data from RCTs to support these recommendations. The study from Kyle et al. mentioned earlier (17), also investigated a subgroup of 35 GCA patients receiving either 40 mg/day or 20 mg/day oral prednisolone. Relapse rate at 2 months was similar in both groups. Besides, there is no evidence supporting any specific GC tapering regimen.

No prospective data are available concerning the use of MP in GCA patients with ischaemic complications. Two trials, however, investigated the value of GC pulse therapy in GCA patients without ischaemic manifestations. The first was a trial on 27 patients receiving either 15 mg/kg/day intravenous MP for 3 days or placebo plus oral GCs. The authors reported a lower cumulative oral GC dose as well as higher remission rates in the MP compared to the control group. The second study investigated 164 uncomplicated GCA patients receiving either 240 mg MP/day for 3 days plus oral GCs or oral GCs alone. No difference between the groups was found regarding cumulative GC dose and discontinuation of GCs.

10.2.2 **When to stop glucocorticoid treatment**

A usual treatment course lasts upwards of 1–2 years. There are, however, patients who require treatment for several years or even indefinitely with GC doses between 1 and 5 mg/day. This is because of relapses occurring as GC dosages are reduced and withdrawn. In general, withdrawal is not possible until patients have had at least 1 year of treatment and have been without clinical and laboratory signs and symptoms of the disease for 2–3 months. It should be noted that despite effective treatment, the majority of patients experience relapses and/or are affected by therapy (particularly GC)-related adverse events.

10.2.3 **Glucocorticoids in relapse treatment**

The reoccurrence of clinical symptoms together with elevations of inflammatory parameters is often seen and indicates a flare of the disease. Under these circumstances, in both PMR and GCA the resumption of GCs at the dose at which control was achieved—and sometimes even at higher dosages—is recommended and mostly is effective. However, sometimes higher dosages are needed to control the disease activity, depending on the intensity of the flare and on the responsibility of

Table 10.1 EULAR evidence-based and consensus-based recommendations on the management of medium to high-dose glucocorticoid therapy in rheumatic diseases

Proposition		SOR		LoE
		VAS; mean (95% CI)	A+B %	
Education and prevention				
1	Explain to patients (and their family and/or carers, including healthcare professionals) the aim of medium/high-dose GC treatment, and the potential risks associated with such therapy	91 (81 to 101)	100	III
2	Discuss measures to mitigate such risks, including diet, regular exercise and appropriate wond care	75 (57 to 93)	75	III/IV
3	Patients with, or at risk of, GC-induced osteoporosis should receive appropriate preventive/therapeutic interventions	91 (84 to 99)	100	I-A
4	Patients and the patients' treatment teams should receive appropriate, practical advice on how to manage with GC-induced hypothalamic-pituitary-adrenal axis suppression	84 (69 to 91)	75	IV
5	Provide an accessible resource to promote best practice in the management of patients using medium/high-dose GCs to general practitioners	80 (69 to 91)	75	IV
Dosing/risk-benefit				
6	Before starting medium/high-dose GC treatment consider comorbidities predisposing to AEs. These include diabetes, glucose intolerance, cardiovascular disease, peptic ulcer disease, recurrent infections, immunosuppression, (risk factors of) glaucoma and osteoporosis. Patients with these comorbidities require tight control to manage the risk/benefit ratio	85 (76 to 94)	83	IV
7	Select the appropriate starting dose to achieve therapeutic response, taking into account the risk of under treatment	85 (76 to 95)	92	I-A/IV
8	Keep the requirement for continuing GC treatment under constant review, and titrate the dose against therapeutic response, risk of under treatment and development of AEs	82 (72 to 94)	92	IV
9	If long-term medium/high-dose GC therapy is anticipated to be necessary. Actively consider GC-sparing therapy	REJECTED		
Monitoring				
10	All patients should have appropriate monitoring for clinically signicant AEs. The treating physician should be aware of the possible occurrence of diabetes, hypertension, weight gain, infections, osteoporotic factures, osteonecrosis, myopathy, eye problems, skin problem, skin problems and neuropsychological AEs	85 (79 to 92)	75	IV

A+B %, percentage, of the task force members that strongly to fully recommended this proposition based on an A–E ordinal scal (A, fully recommended, B, strongly recommended); AEs, adverse effects; CI, confidence interval; GC, glucocorticoid; LoE, level of evidence; SOR, Strength of recommendation; VAS, visual analogue scale (0–100 mm 0= not recommended at all, 100, fully recommended.)

Reproduced from Annals of the Rheumatic Diseases, EULAR evidence-based and consensus-based recommendations on the management of medium to high-dose glucocorticoid therapy in rheumatic diseases, N Duru et al, 2013; 72(12):1905–1913 with permission from BMJ Publishing Group Ltd.

the individual patient. This re-increase of the GC dose should usually be followed by a slower tapering (smaller decrements and/or longer intervals for the reduction steps), especially in those patients who experience several relapses of the disease. GCA-type relapses (headache, jaw pain, or ischaemic symptoms) should be treated by appropriate high-dose GCs.

10.3 **How to achieve a proper benefit to risk ratio when using glucocorticoids**

The key approach for a reasonable and successful systematic GC treatment is to minimize the dose of the administered GC in order to reduce the occurrence of adverse effects according to the principle 'as much as necessary, but as little as possible' (21, 22). The 2007 recommendations of the EULAR GC task force on the proper use of systemic GCs in rheumatic diseases such as PMR and GCA also comprise the thorough discussion of potential adverse effects of GCs with the patient, and the evaluation and treatment (where indicated) of comorbidities and risk factors, for these adverse effects are key measures (22). Furthermore, monitoring for body weight, blood pressure, peripheral oedema, cardiac insufficiency, serum lipids, blood and/or urine glucose, ocular pressure depending on individual patient' risk, GC dose, and GC duration is suggested (22). Also, recommendations for the prevention and treatment of GC-induced osteoporosis should be followed (22). The overarching principles of the EULAR/ACR PMR guidelines stress the importance of assessing risk factors for common GC adverse effects (e.g. diabetes, osteoporosis, hypertension, and glaucoma) in the choice of individualized GC doses in PMR.

Very recently, the EULAR GC task force has developed evidence-based and consensus-based recommendations to assist clinicians with balancing the risks and benefits when treating rheumatic diseases with medium- to high-dose GCs (which apply particularly to GCA patients) (23). These updated recommendations are (a) based on the most recent literature, (b) also address the use of higher GC dosages to make them more broadly applicable and (c) now cover education and prevention, dosing, risks/benefits, and monitoring. The respective recommendations are given in Table 10.1.

10.4 **Conclusion**

GCs form the mainstay of therapy for PMR and GCA since they exert strong anti-inflammatory and immunosuppressive effects. There are different views on how to initiate and taper the GC therapy, but the differences are rather subtle and do not represent a serious problem in daily clinical practice. Most important is to follow recently updated recommendations on how to achieve a good benefit to risk ratio when using GCs.

References

1. Buttgereit F, Saag KG, Cutolo M, et al. The molecular basis for the effectiveness, toxicity, and resistance to glucocorticoids: focus on the treatment of rheumatoid arthritis. Scan J Rheumatol 2005; 34(1):14–21.

2. Buttgereit F, Straub RH, Wehling M, et al. Glucocorticoids in the treatment of rheumatic diseases: an update on the mechanisms of action. Arthritis Rheum 2004; 50(11):3408–17.

3. Schacke H, Docke WD, Asadullah K. Mechanisms involved in the side effects of glucocorticoids. Pharmacol Ther 2002; 96(1):23–43.

4. Stahn C, Buttgereit F. Genomic and nongenomic effects of glucocorticoids. Nat Clin Pract Rheumatol 2008; 4(10):525–33.

5. Schacke H, Schottelius A, Docke WD, et al. Dissociation of transactivation from transrepression by a selective glucocorticoid receptor agonist leads to separation of therapeutic effects from side effects. Proc Natl Acad Sci U S A 2004; 101(1):227–32.

6. Song IH, Gold R, Straub RH, et al. New glucocorticoids on the horizon: repress, don't activate! J Rheumatol 2005; 32(7):1199–207.

7. Strehl C, Buttgereit F. Optimized glucocorticoid therapy: teaching old drugs new tricks. Mol Cell Endocrinol 2013; 380(1–2):32–40.

8. Buttgereit F, Scheffold A. Rapid glucocorticoid effects on immune cells. Steroids 2002; 67(6):529–34.

9. Falkenstein E, Norman AW, Wehling M. Mannheim classification of nongenomically initiated (rapid) steroid action(s). J Clin Endocrinol Metab 2000; 85(5):2072–5.

10. Croxtall JD, Choudhury Q, Flower RJ. Glucocorticoids act within minutes to inhibit recruitment of signalling factors to activated EGF receptors through a receptor-dependent, transcription-independent mechanism. Br J Pharmacol 2000; 130(2):289–98.

11. Cato AC, Nestl A, Mink S. Rapid actions of steroid receptors in cellular signaling pathways. Sci STKE 2002; 2002(138):RE9.

12. Hafezi-Moghadam A, Simoncini T, Yang Z, et al. Acute cardiovascular protective effects of corticosteroids are mediated by non-transcriptional activation of endothelial nitric oxide synthase. Nat Med 2002; 8(5):473–9.

13. Lee SR, Kim HK, Youm JB, et al. Non-genomic effect of glucocorticoids on cardiovascular system. Pflugers Arch 2012; 464(6):549–59.

14. Dejaco C, Singh YP, Perel P, et al. Recommendations for management of polymyalgia rheumatica: a European League Against Rheumatism and American College of Rheumatology collaborative initiative. Ann Rheum Dis 2015; 74(10):1799–1806.

15. Dasgupta B, Borg FA, Hassan N, et al. BSR and BHPR guidelines for the management of polymyalgia rheumatica. Rheumatology 2010; 49(1):186–90.

16. Eizenga WH, Hakvoort L, Dubbeld P, et al. [Dutch College of General Practitioner's practice guideline on polymyalgia rheumatica and temporal arteritis]. Nederlands tijdschrift voor geneeskunde 2010; 154:A1919.

17. Kyle V, Hazleman BL. Treatment of polymyalgia rheumatica and giant cell arteritis. I. Steroid regimens in the first two months. Ann Rheum Dis 1989; 48(8):658–61.

18. Kremers HM, Reinalda MS, Crowson CS, et al. Relapse in a population based cohort of patients with polymyalgia rheumatica. J Rheumatol 2005; 32:65–73.

19. Dolan AL, Moniz C, Dasgupta B, et al. Effects of inflammation and treatment on bone turnover and bone mass in polymyalgia rheumatica. Arthritis Rheum 1997; 40(11):2022–9.

20. Dasgupta B, Dolan AL, Panayi GS, et al. An initially double-blind controlled 96 week trial of depot methylprednisolone against oral prednisolone in the treatment of polymyalgia rheumatica. Br J Rheumatol 1998; 37(2):189–95.

21. Buttgereit F, Burmester GR, Lipworth BJ. Optimised glucocorticoid therapy: the sharpening of an old spear. Lancet 2005; 365(9461):801–3.

22. Hoes JN, Jacobs JW, Boers M, et al. EULAR evidence-based recommendations on the management of systemic glucocorticoid therapy in rheumatic diseases. Ann Rheum Dis 2007; 66(12):1560–7.

23. Duru N, van der Goes MC, Jacobs JW, et al. EULAR evidence-based and consensus-based recommendations on the management of medium to high-dose glucocorticoid therapy in rheumatic diseases. Ann Rheum Dis 2013; 72(12):1905–13.

Chapter 11

Role of steroid-sparing agents

Christian Dejaco

Key points

- Methotrexate was effective as a steroid-sparing agent in randomized controlled trials in polymyalgia rheumatica (PMR) and giant cell arteritis (GCA).
- Data on second-line conventional disease-modifying anti-rheumatic drugs are scarce, leflunomide and azathioprine may be effective.
- The value of biological agents for the treatment of PMR and GCA is unclear. Tumour necrosis factor-alpha antagonists were not effective in randomized controlled trials. Case series on tocilizumab are promising.

11.1 Introduction

The course of PMR and GCA is variable: some patients receive glucocorticoids (GCs) for a period of 1–2 years, whereas others require treatment for several years, suffering frequent relapses and high cumulative GC doses (1). The prevalence of GC-induced adverse events is high, affecting up to 50% and 86% of PMR and GCA patients, respectively (2, 3). Therefore, GC-sparing agents are needed, at least for those patients with the highest risk for GC side effects.

As detailed in Table 11.1 and the following paragraphs, most evidence is available for methotrexate (MTX) as a GC-sparing agent in PMR and GCA, whereas other conventional disease-modifying anti-rheumatic drugs (DMARDs) have been studied occasionally. Concerning biological DMARDs, most data are available for tumour necrosis factor alpha (TNFα) blocking agents and tocilizumab.

11.2 Methotrexate as a steroid-sparing agent

11.2.1 Methotrexate in addition to glucocorticoids for treatment of polymyalgia rheumatica

The new 2015 European League Against Rheumatism/American College of Rheumatology (EULAR/ACR) guidelines for the management of PMR recommend considering MTX in new PMR patients with an increased risk for relapses and/or risk factors for GC-induced adverse events (see Table 11.2 for risk factors). In addition, MTX may be used in patients with established PMR who have either relapsed (on or

Table 11.1 Disease-modifying anti-rheumatic drugs for treatment of PMR and/or GCA

Substance	Disease	Drug dose	Suggested indication	Evidence
Conventional DMARDs				
Methotrexate	PMR GCA	7.5–10 mg/ week 7.5–15 mg/ week	*1st-line DMARD in new PMR or GCA patients* with risk factors for relapses and/or pro- longed therapy as well as for GC-related side effects *Relapsing patients*	4 RCTs for PMR (6–10) and 3 RCTs for GCA (13–15) (variable quality, best studies indicate benefit of MTX)
Azathioprine	PMR/ GCA	100–150 mg/ day	*2nd-line DMARD in PMR or GCA patients* unable to reduce GC dose/GC side effects	1 low-quality RCT (17)
Leflunomide	PMR/ GCA	10–20 mg/ day	*2nd-line DMARD in PMR or GCA patients* unable to reduce GC dose/GC side effects	Case series (21, 22)
Cyclophosphamide	GCA	500–1000 mg IV pulses (1 pulse/ month)	*>2nd-line DMARD in GCA patients* unable to reduce GC dose/GC side effects *Life-threatening GCA*	Case series (23)
Mycophenolate	GCA	1000–2000 mg/day	*>2nd-line DMARD in GCA patients* unable to reduce GC dose/GC side effects	Case report (24)
Ciclosporin	PMR/ GCA	n.a.	*Not useful in PMR/GCA* due to toxicity and due to lack of benefit	2 low-quality RCTs (18, 19)
Dapsone	GCA	n.a.	*Not useful in GCA due* to toxicity and minimal benefit	1 low-quality RCT (20)
Biological agents				
Tocilizumab	PMR/ GCA	8 mg/kg body weight	*2nd-line DMARD in PMR or GCA patients* unable to reduce GC dose/GC side effects	Case series (36–38)
Anakinra	GCA	100 mg/day	*> 2nd-line DMARD in PMR or GCA patients* unable to reduce GC dose/GC side effects	Case report (35)
Rituximab	GCA	1000 mg on days 1+15	*> 2nd-line DMARD in PMR or GCA patients* unable to reduce GC dose/GC side effects	Case report (41, 42)

(continued)

Table 11.1 Continued				
TNFα blockers	PMR GCA	n.a.	*Not recommended in PMR or GCA due to lack of benefit*	1 high-quality trial on infliximab each in PMR and GCA (30, 34); 1 moderate and 1 low-quality trial on etanercept in PMR and GCA (31, 33), respectively; 1 moderate quality trial on adalimumab in GCA (32)

DMARD, disease-modifying anti-rheumatic drug; GC, glucocorticoid; GCA, giant cell arteritis; IV; intravenous; MTX, methotrexate; n.a., not applicable; PMR, polymyalgia rheumatica; RCT, randomized controlled trial.

PMR/GCA indicates that PMR and GCA were studied as a single group; PMR and GCA on two separate lines indicates that studies are available for both PMR and GCA.

off GCs), have an inadequate response to GCs, or experienced GC-related adverse events. In all these cases, MTX may be applied in addition to standard GC treatment at a dose of 7.5–10 mg/week. The efficacy and safety of higher MTX doses in PMR is elusive so far.

The British Society of Rheumatology (BSR) recommendations suggest using MTX in relapsing patients (after the second relapse) and the guidelines of the German Society of Internal Medicine recommend MTX for patients unable to reduce the GC dose below 10 mg/day (4, 5).

The efficacy of MTX was studied in four randomized controlled trials with variable quality (ranging from very low to high) and yielding discordant results. Those trials demonstrating a benefit of MTX over placebo regarding relapse rate, cumulative GC dose, and other outcomes were generally of a higher quality than studies reporting no effect of MTX (6–10). This result and the enormous experience with MTX from other inflammatory rheumatic diseases (and thus its well-known safety profile) justify the

Table 11.2 Possible risk factors for relapses and/or prolonged therapy as well as for glucocorticoid related side effects	
Risk factors for relapse/ prolonged therapy	**Risk factors for glucocorticoid-related side effects**
Female sex High ESR (>40 mm/1st hour) Peripheral inflammatory arthritis	Female sex Comorbidities: Hypertension Diabetes, glucose intolerance Cardiovascular disease Dyslipidaemia Peptic ulcer Osteoporosis Cataract (Risk factors of) glaucoma Chronic or recurrent infections Co-medication with NSAIDs

ESR, erythrocyte sedimentation rate; NSAIDs, non-steroidal anti-inflammatory drugs.

consideration of MTX as a steroid-sparing agent in new and established PMR patients at an increased risk for a worse outcome.

11.2.2 Methotrexate in addition to glucocorticoids for treatment of giant cell arteritis

The 2009 EULAR guidelines for management of GCA recommend considering MTX as an adjunctive therapy to GCs in each GCA patient (11). Similarly, the BSR guidelines discuss the value of an early application of MTX treatment in GCA and further emphasize that MTX should be prescribed to cases with relapsing disease (particularly after the second relapse) (12). The German Society of Internal Medicine recommends the introduction of MTX in GCA patients whose GC dose cannot be reduced below 10 mg/day.

Three randomized controlled trials were conducted to test the efficacy of MTX at doses ranging from 7.5 to 15 mg/week (13–15). Two of these studies with low (13) and moderate (15) quality reported no benefit of MTX over placebo concerning relapses, treatment duration, and cumulative GC dose, whereas one high-quality study observed a shortening of GC treatment duration and a reduction of the cumulative GC dose in the MTX group (14). A meta-analysis pooling the original data of these three trials found a significant benefit of MTX regarding the risk of the first relapse and the cumulative GC dose; however, the 95% confidence interval of the overall effect was close to the null effect (16). In addition, methodological weaknesses of the original studies such as the unclear handling of missing data and the recalculation of the power analysis in the trial by Hoffman et al. (15) raises further concerns about the validity of this meta-analysis. The early application of MTX in GCA (particularly in patients at risk) is nevertheless reasonable, given the high prevalence of GC-related adverse events (affecting up to 86% of patients), the assumed effect of MTX as a steroid-sparing agent, and the good safety profile of the drug (2). MTX was well tolerated in all randomized trials mentioned, with only a slightly higher rate of adverse events in the intervention compared to the control groups.

11.3 Value of non-methotrexate conventional DMARDs

Only low-quality trials have examined non-MTX conventional DMARDs in PMR and GCA. Azathioprine was tested in 31 patients with PMR and/or GCA (both conditions were considered as a single disease) with stable remission while taking oral prednisone at a dose of greater than 5 mg daily (17). After 52 weeks, the cumulative GC dose was lower in the azathioprine group; however, the trial suffered from a high drop-out rate (one-third of all patients), and the handling of missing data was unclear. Ciclosporin was studied in two open randomized trials in GCA (one of these also included PMR patients) yielding no benefit of the substance (18, 19). The drug, however, was associated with an unacceptably high rate of adverse events (19). In another open randomized trial, dapsone showed a moderate benefit regarding relapse rate; however, the prevalence of haematological complications was unacceptably high (20).

Several drugs were used in small case series of PMR and GCA. Among these, promising results were reported for leflunomide regarding both PMR and GCA (21, 22). Cyclophosphamide may be an option for GCA patients with life-threatening manifestations or in case of GC dependency, severe GC side effects, and failure of other conventional immunosuppressive agents (23). Mycophenolate mofetil was used in three cases with GCA, yielding a good clinical effect and tolerability (24).

11.4 Biological agents

The 2015 EULAR/ACR guidelines for the management of PMR, the 2009 EULAR recommendations on GCA, and the BSR guidelines on GCA all discourage the use of anti-TNFα agents for the treatment of PMR and GCA. Although initial case reports, case series, and small open label studies were promising (25–29), subsequent randomized controlled trials did not confirm a benefit of TNFα blockers for treatment of PMR or GCA.

In PMR, infliximab was studied in 51 patients in a placebo-controlled trial over 52 weeks (30). Infliximab was applied to new patients in addition to a standard GC regimen; however, no benefit was observed regarding primary and secondary outcome parameters. Etanercept was compared with placebo in a 2-week study in a total of 22 patients (31). None of these patients received GCs. Etanercept was not superior to placebo in this study.

For GCA, adalimumab, etanercept, and infliximab were each studied in one randomized controlled trial (32–34). The adalimumab trial was stopped early because of an insufficient recruitment (after 70% of the projected patients were included) (32). The authors found no difference between adalimumab and placebo regarding any of the outcomes investigated. However, a type II error cannot be excluded due to the low recruitment rate. The infliximab study was also terminated earlier because it became evident after an interim analysis that the substance was not effective (34). Etanercept was studied in a small randomized trial in patients with established, stable disease while taking prednisone at a dose of 10 mg or higher daily. A lower cumulative GC dose was found in the etanercept group whereas no significant difference was found regarding any of the other efficacy parameters. This study was also terminated earlier and only 6/17 patients completed the first 12 months (33).

Other biological agents that were used in small case series of GCA and/or PMR are the interleukin (IL)-1 receptor antagonist anakinra and the IL-6 receptor antibody tocilizumab (35–38). The blockade of these cytokines might be promising given that IL-6 is increased in the plasma of PMR patients and IL-1 beta and IL-6 were elevated in plasma and inflamed tissue of GCA patients (39).

Anakinra was used effectively in three patients with GCA, yielding an improvement of symptoms and inflammatory biomarkers (35). For tocilizumab, several case reports and case series are available (as monotherapy or in combination with GCs), all suggesting a good efficacy of this drug in PMR and GCA (36–38). Currently, tocilizumab is being studied in a multicentre randomized controlled trial ('GiACTA') in patients with new or relapsing GCA (40). This trial will enrol 250 patients and is designed as a 52-week blinded study followed by a 104 weeks of open-label extension.

Notably, a few case reports suggested a benefit of rituximab for treatment of GCA, although there is no definite role of B cells in the pathogenesis of the disease (41–43).

References

1. Weyand CM, Fulbright JW, Evans JM, et al. Corticosteroid requirements in polymyalgia rheumatica. Arch Intern Med 1999; 159:577–84.

2. Proven A, Gabriel SE, Orces C, et al. Glucocorticoid therapy in giant cell arteritis: duration and adverse outcomes. *Arthritis Rheum* 2003; 49:703–8.

3. Dejaco C, Duftner C, Dasgupta B, et al. Polymyalgia rheumatica and giant cell arteritis: management of two diseases of the elderly. *Aging Health* 2011;7:633–45.

4. Dasgupta B, Borg FA, Hassan N, et al. BSR and BHPR guidelines for the management of polymyalgia rheumatica. Rheumatology *(Oxford)* 2010; 49(1):186–90.

5. Dasgupta B, Borg FA, Hassan N, et al. BSR and BHPR guidelines for the management of giant cell arteritis. *Rheumatology (Oxford)* 2010; 49(8):1594–7.

6. Mukhtyar C, Guillevin L, Cid MC, et al. EULAR recommendations for the management of large vessel vasculitis. *Ann Rheum Dis* 2009; 68:318–23.

7. Schmidt WA, Gromnica Ihle E. Polymyalgia rheumatica und Riesenzellarteriitis (Arteriitis temporalis). In Busse O, Fleig W, Mayet W, et al. (eds) *Rationelle Diagnostik und Therapie in der Inneren Medizin: Leitlinien-basierte Empfehlungen für die Prax.* Elsevier Inc, 2011: Chapter 5.2.

8. Ferraccioli G, Salaffi F, De Vita S, et al. Methotrexate in polymyalgia rheumatica: preliminary results of an open, randomized study. *J Rheumatol* 1996; 23:624–8.

9. Nazarinia AM, Moghimi J, Toussi J. Efficacy of methotrexate in patients with polymyalgia rheumatica. *Koomesh* 2012; 14:265–70.

10. Van der Veen MJ, Dinant HJ, van Booma-Frankfort C, et al. Can methotrexate be used as a steroid sparing agent in the treatment of polymyalgia rheumatica and giant cell arteritis? (Erratum appears in *Ann Rheum Dis* 1996; 55(8):563). *Ann Rheum Dis* 1996; 55:218–23.

11. Caporali R, Cimmino MA, Ferraccioli G, et al. Prednisone plus methotrexate for polymyalgia rheumatica: a randomized, double-blind, placebo-controlled trial. *Ann Intern Med* 2004; 141:493–500.

12. Lee JH, Choi ST, Kim JS, et al. Clinical characteristics and prognostic factors for relapse in patients with polymyalgia rheumatica (PMR). *Rheumatol Int* 2013; 33:1475–80.

13. Spiera RF, Mitnick HJ, Kupersmith M, et al. A prospective, double-blind, randomized, placebo controlled trial of methotrexate in the treatment of giant cell arteritis (GCA). *Clin Exp Rheumatol* 2001; 19:495–501.

14. Jover JA, Hernández-García C, Morado IC, et al. Combined treatment of giant-cell arteritis with methotrexate and prednisone. a randomized, double-blind, placebo-controlled trial. *Ann Intern Med* 2001; 134:106–14.

15. Hoffman GS, Cid MC, Hellmann DB, et al. A multicenter, randomized, double-blind, placebo-controlled trial of adjuvant methotrexate treatment for giant cell arteritis. *Arthritis Rheum* 2002; 46:1309–18.

16. Mahr AD, Jover JA, Spiera RF, et al. Adjunctive methotrexate for treatment of giant cell arteritis: an individual patient data meta-analysis. *Arthritis Rheum* 2007; 56:2789–97.

17. De Silva M, Hazleman BL. Azathioprine in giant cell arteritis/polymyalgia rheumatica: a double-blind study. *Ann Rheum Dis* 1986; 45:136–8.

18. Schaufelberger C, Andersson R, Nordborg E. No additive effect of cyclosporin A compared with glucocorticoid treatment alone in giant cell arteritis: results of an open, controlled, randomized study. *Br J Rheumatol* 1998; 37:464–5.

19. Schaufelberger C, Möllby H, Uddhammar A, et al. No additional steroid-sparing effect of cyclosporine A in giant cell arteritis. *Scand J Rheumatol* 2006; 35:327–9.

20. Liozon F, Vidal E, Barrier J-H. Dapsone in giant cell arteritis treatment. *Eur J Intern Med* 1993; 4:207–14.

21. Diamantopoulos AP, Hetland H, Myklebust G. Leflunomide as a corticosteroid-sparing agent in giant cell arteritis and polymyalgia rheumatica: a case series. *Biomed Res Int* 2013; 2013:120638.

22. Adizie T, Christidis D, Dharmapaliah C, et al. Efficacy and tolerability of leflunomide in difficult-to-treat polymyalgia rheumatica and giant cell arteritis: a case series. *Int J Clin Pract* 2012 ; 66:906–9.

23. De Boysson H, Boutemy J, Creveuil C, et al. Is there a place for cyclophosphamide in the treatment of giant-cell arteritis? A case series and systematic review. *Semin Arthritis Rheum* 2013; 43:105–12.

24. Sciascia S, Piras D, Baldovino S, et al. Mycophenolate mofetil as steroid-sparing treatment for elderly patients with giant cell arteritis: report of three cases. *Aging Clin Exp Res* 2012 ; 24:273–7.

25. Aikawa NE, Pereira RMR, Lage L, et al. Anti-TNF therapy for polymyalgia rheumatica: report of 99 cases and review of the literature. *Clin Rheumatol* 2012; 31:575–9.

26. Catanoso MG, Macchioni P, Boiardi L, et al. Treatment of refractory polymyalgia rheumatica with etanercept: an open pilot study. *Arthritis Rheum* 2007; 57:1514–19.

27. Ahmed MM, Mubashir E, Hayat S, et al. Treatment of refractory temporal arteritis with adalimumab. *Clin Rheumatol* 2007; 26:1353–5.

28. Airò P, Antonioli CM, Vianelli M, et al. Anti-tumour necrosis factor treatment with infliximab in a case of giant cell arteritis resistant to steroid and immunosuppressive drugs. *Rheumatology (Oxford)* 2002; 41:347–9.

29. Tan AL, Holdsworth J, Pease C, et al. Successful treatment of resistant giant cell arteritis with etanercept. *Ann Rheum Dis* 2003; 62:373–4.

30. Salvarani C, Macchioni P, Manzini C, et al. Infliximab plus prednisone or placebo plus prednisone for the initial treatment of polymyalgia rheumatica: a randomized trial. *Ann Intern Med* 2007; 146(9):631–9.

31. Kreiner F, Galbo H. Effect of etanercept in polymyalgia rheumatica: a randomized controlled trial. *Arthritis Res Ther* 2010; 12:R176.

32. Seror R, Baron G, Hachulla E, et al. Adalimumab for steroid sparing in patients with giant-cell arteritis: results of a multicentre randomised controlled trial. *Ann Rheum Dis* 2013; 73:2074–81.

33. Martínez-Taboada VM, Rodríguez-Valverde V, Carreño L, et al. A double-blind placebo controlled trial of etanercept in patients with giant cell arteritis and corticosteroid side effects. *Ann Rheum Dis* 2008; 67:625–30.

34. Hoffman GS, Cid MC, Rendt-Zagar KE, et al. Infliximab for maintenance of glucocorticosteroid-induced remission of giant cell arteritis: a randomized trial. *Ann Intern Med* 2007; 146:621–30.

35. Ly K-H, Stirnemann J, Liozon E, et al. Interleukin-1 blockade in refractory giant cell arteritis. *Joint Bone Spine* 2014; 81:76–8.

36. Macchioni P, Boiardi L, Catanoso M, et al. Tocilizumab for polymyalgia rheumatica: report of two cases and review of the literature. *Semin Arthritis Rheum* 2013; 43:113–18.

37. Osman M, Pagnoux C, Dryden DM, et al. The role of biological agents in the management of large vessel vasculitis (LVV): a systematic review and meta-analysis. *PLoS One* 2014; 9:e115026.

38. Loricera J, Blanco R, Castañeda S, et al. Tocilizumab in refractory aortitis: study on 16 patients and literature review. *Clin Exp Rheumatol*; 32 Suppl 8:79–89.

39. Martinez-Taboada VM, Alvarez L, RuizSoto M, et al. Giant cell arteritis and polymyalgia rheumatica: role of cytokines in the pathogenesis and implications for treatment. *Cytokine* 2008; 44:207–20.

40. Unizony SH, Dasgupta B, Fisheleva E, et al. Design of the tocilizumab in giant cell arteritis trial. *Int J Rheumatol* 2013; 2013:912562.

41. Bhatia A, Ell PJ, Edwards JCW. Anti-CD20 monoclonal antibody (rituximab) as an adjunct in the treatment of giant cell arteritis. *Ann Rheum Dis* 2005; 64:1099–100.

42. Mayrbaeurl B, Hinterreiter M, Burgstaller S, et al. The first case of a patient with neutropenia and giant-cell arteritis treated with rituximab. *Clin Rheumatol* 2007; 26:1597–8.

43. Weyand CM, Goronzy JJ. Immune mechanisms in medium and large-vessel vasculitis. *Nat Rev Rheumatol* 2013; 9:731–40.

Chapter 12

Treatment of a relapse and approach to difficult-to-treat patients

Bhaskar Dasgupta

Key points

- Early correct assessment of polymyalgia rheumatica (PMR) and giant cell arteritis (GCA) is essential for prevention of flares and difficult-to-treat disease. The terminology 'atypical' PMR or GCA should be discouraged.
- The assessment should involve risk stratification considering factors such as demographics, disease severity, co-morbidities, and risk factors for glucocorticoid (GC)-related adverse events.
- Disease-modifying antirheumatic drugs (DMARDs) such as methotrexate should be introduced early if GC therapy alone is considered insufficient or potentially toxic.
- Clinical trials are ongoing to identify more effective biological (such as tocilizumab) and non-biological DMARDs (such as leflunomide) in PMR and GCA.

12.1 Introduction

Optimal treatment of PMR and GCA and prevention of flares and complications begins with correct assessment of the patient at presentation. Although GCA at presentation requires immediate high-dose GCs to prevent ischaemic complications, short- and long-term management of both diseases should be predicated to careful case ascertainment and even more careful risk stratification. This is the ethos of the European League Against Rheumatism/American College of Rheumatology (EULAR/ACR) PMR guidelines (1), which also apply to the updated BSR GCA guidelines under development.

With PMR, the task begins with a holistic evaluation upfront with exclusion of mimicking conditions. A safe and specific approach is advocated for the accurate assessment of PMR as detailed in Chapter 9. This will allow early specialist referral for diagnostic conundrums before they present as crises or flares.

The 2015 EULAR/ACR collaborative PMR recommendations (1) emphasize an individualized management approach that strikes the balance between efficacy and undesirable effects of GC therapy while taking into account coexisting co-morbidities that may interact with disease and/or treatment.

The practice of defining patients, who do not respond to GCs as 'atypical PMR', is discouraged. This results in delayed diagnosis of serious conditions (such as cancer, bacterial endocarditis, or a primary systemic vasculitis), increases referrals for 'flares' of suspected PMR, as well as incorrect overtreatment of many non-inflammatory conditions such as osteoarthritis, rotator cuff problems, or fibromyalgia. As the 2012 PMR classification criteria highlight, 'steroid responsiveness' should be discouraged as a diagnostic test since it can be a pitfall for treatment of both conditions (2).

Initial relapses may be treated by returning to previous higher GC doses or by single injections of depot methylprednisolone. The 2015 PMR guidelines allow introduction of methotrexate (MTX) as early as 4 weeks for patients with severe disease, peripheral arthritis, and risks for prolonged GC therapy (1). A meta-analysis of MTX in GCA at a dose of 10–15 mg/week versus placebo in 166 patients showed an effect in reducing relapse rate and lowering the cumulative dose of GC therapy in GCA (3). MTX therapy has also been shown to be associated with a higher probability of achieving sustained discontinuation of corticosteroids for 24 or more weeks (hazard ratio 2.84, p = 0.001) (3). Also, the rates of first relapse of cranial signs and symptoms at 48 weeks were 40% (95% confidence interval (CI) 28–51%) among the MTX group and 47% (95% CI 34–59%) among the placebo group. Overall, high-quality studies suggest a benefit of early introduction of MTX for treatment of PMR and GCA whereas negative trials were generally of lower quality. The addition of MTX to GCs should therefore be considered on an individual basis in patients at high risk for GC adverse events, relapsing disease, and/or prolonged GC therapy (Figure 12.1).

There is clearly an unmet need for more effective and safer disease-modifying therapy for both PMR and GCA. Leflunomide may be an effective corticosteroid-sparing agent in patients with difficult-to-treat GCA and two case series showed either a partial or complete response and leflunomide was well tolerated (4, 5). Randomized controlled trials (RCTs) of leflunomide in both PMR and GCA are required. Mycophenolate mofetil has been effective in a case series of three elderly GCA patients at high risk of long-term, high-dose GCs due to comorbidities (6). Cyclophosphamide, both as monthly pulses and orally, has been demonstrated to be efficacious in GCA patients who are GC dependent or who have a high risk of GC-related adverse effects although this is at the expense of significant adverse effects (7). Azathioprine has been shown in a single RCT to lower daily prednisolone dose whereas ciclosporin and dapsone have not been associated with significant beneficial effects despite considerable toxicity.

12.2 **Biological therapies**

Although initial reports suggested the efficacy of tumour necrosis factor alpha inhibition (8), this was not replicated in RCTs (9–11). Infliximab, etanercept, and adalimumab all have failed to meet their primary efficacy outcomes in GCA.

There are many case reports and series of efficacious and safe interleukin (IL)-6R blockade with tocilizumab (TCZ) in refractory and relapsing cases of GCA, PMR, and large-vessel vasculitis (12–14). GC-free clinical and imaging remission could be achieved with continuous therapy although relapses were common after dose tapering or stopping TCZ. The ongoing GiACTA RCT (15) seeks to compare efficacy and safety of subcutaneous TCZ 162 mg weekly and twice weekly with placebo, with all three arms aiming to taper off GCs in 6 months. This is also compared with a 'standard of care'

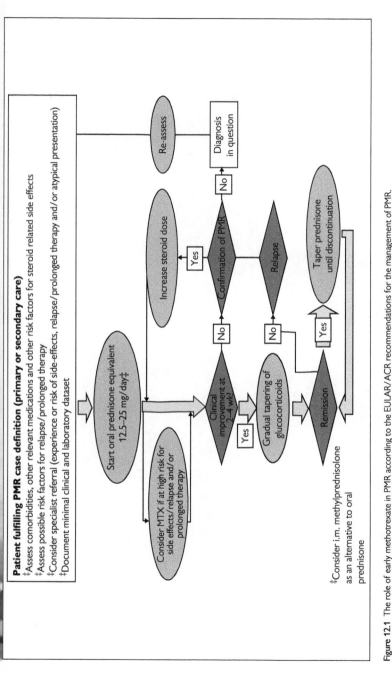

Figure 12.1 The role of early methotrexate in PMR according to the EULAR/ACR recommendations for the management of PMR.

Reproduced from Christian Dejaco et al, 2015 Recommendations for the Management of Polymyalgia Rheumatica: A European League Against Rheumatism/American College of Rheumatology Collaborative Initiative, September 2015, with permission from Wiley.

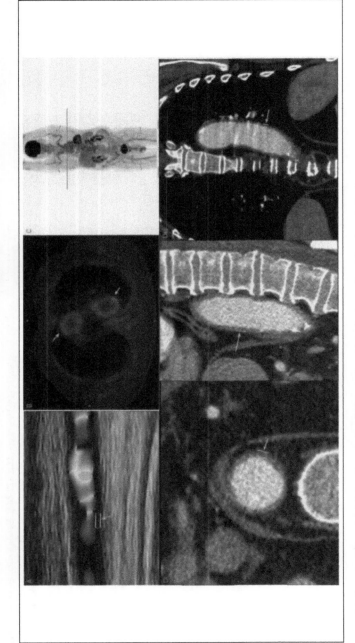

Figure 12.2 (See colour plate section). Polymyalgia arteritica: GCA presenting with predominant polymyalgia and constitutional symptoms.

arm of oral GC taper over 12 months. The trial has completed recruitment and results awaited in late 2016.

Successful IL-1 blockade using anakinra in three cases demonstrated improvement in biochemical markers and/or symptoms: two of the three had improvement in terms of imaging with the loss of arterial inflammation using fluorodeoxyglucose (FDG)-positron emission tomography (PET) following anakinra (16). Gevokizumab (GVK), a monoclonal antibody to IL-1 beta, is currently being trialled in relapsing GCA with polymyalgic or systemic symptoms (Figure 12.2). The primary outcome at 4 weeks aims to achieve complete response without increased GC dose after two fortnightly injections of GVK versus placebo.

Targeting IL-23 is a conceptually interesting possibility, given the pivotal role of this cytokine in T-helper 17 cell differentiation (17), as well as targeting IL-17 itself, due to the importance of this T-cell subset in the genesis of GCA. A triple-arm RCT of single infusions of secukinumab (anti-IL-17) and canakinumab (anti-IL-1) versus placebo GC in newly diagnosed GC-naïve PMR showed a significant effect in both biological arms although this was not comparable to the GC response. However, there was evidence of GC sparing in both biological arms (18).

Rituximab (anti-B cell) has been used successfully in abdominal aortitis and large-vessel vasculitis with/without retroperitoneal fibrosis, a plasma cell-mediated and immunoglobulin G4-related disease (19). There is a case report of rituximab used as an adjunct during therapy of a patient with GCA and PMR with reversal of vascular uptake of FDG in external carotid and subclavian arteries, as well as part of the abdominal aorta and both iliac arteries, using FDG-PET (20). Rituximab has also been reported as effective in a patient with temporal arteritis associated with neutropenia (21).

Blocking CD28-mediated T-cell co-stimulation with abatacept is currently being tested in a multicentre trial in large-vessel vasculitis (Abatacept in GCA and Takayasu's arteritis (AGATA)). Targeting other cell–T-cell interactions may also become feasible, including notch-induced differentiation, and natural killer receptor function.

The use of kinase inhibition to target downstream pathways from receptor ligation has been successful in other diseases, and downstream targets including ROCK may become a therapeutic option. In one *in vitro* analysis, imatinib effectively suppressed platelet-derived growth factor signalling in myointimal cells cultured from temporal artery biopsies resulting in reduced cell outgrowth (22).

References

1. Dejaco C, Singh, YP, Perel, P et al. 2015 Recommendations for the management of polymyalgia rheumatica: a European League Against Rheumatism/American College of Rheumatology collaborative initiative. Ann Rheum Dis 2015; 74(10):1799–807.

2. Dasgupta B, Cimmino MA, Maradit-Kremers H, et al. 2012 provisional classification criteria for polymyalgia rheumatica: a European League Against Rheumatism/American College of Rheumatology collaborative initiative. Ann Rheum Dis 2012; 71(4):484–92.

3. Mahr AD, Jover JA, Spiera RF, et al. Adjunctive methotrexate for treatment of giant cell arteritis: an individual patient data meta-analysis. Arthritis Rheum 2007; 56(8):2789–97.

4. Adizie T, Christidis D, Dharmapaliah C, et al. Efficacy and tolerability of leflunomide in difficult-to-treat polymyalgia rheumatica and giant cell arteritis: a case series. Int J Clin Pract 2012; 66(9):906–9.

5. Diamantopoulos AP, Hetland H, Myklebust G. Leflunomide as a corticosteroid-sparing agent in giant cell arteritis and polymyalgia rheumatica: a case series. BioMed Res Int 2013; 2013:120638.

6. Sciascia S, Piras D, Baldovino S, *et al*. Mycophenolate mofetil as steroid-sparing treatment for elderly patients with giant cell arteritis: report of three cases. *Aging Clin Exp Res* 2012; 24(3):273–7.

7. Loock J, Henes J, Kötter I, *et al*. Treatment of refractory giant cell arteritis with cyclophosphamide: a retrospective analysis of 35 patients from three centres. *Clin Exp Rheumatol* 2012; 30(1 Suppl 70):S70–6.

8. Ahmed MM, Mubashir E, Hayat S, *et al*. Treatment of refractory temporal arteritis with adalimumab. *Clin Rheumatol* 2007; 26(8):1353–5.

9. Hoffman GS, Cid MC, Rendt-Zagar KE, *et al*. Infliximab for maintenance of glucocorticosteroid-induced remission of giant cell arteritis: a randomized trial. *Ann Intern Med* 2007; 146(9):621–30.

10. Martínez-Taboada VM, Rodríguez-Valverde V, Carreño L, *et al*. A double-blind placebo controlled trial of etanercept in patients with giant cell arteritis and corticosteroid side effects. *Ann Rheum Dis* 2008; 67(5):625–30.

11. Seror R, Baron G, Hachulla E, *et al*. Adalimumab for steroid sparing in patients with giant-cell arteritis: results of a multicentre randomised controlled trial. *Ann Rheum Dis* 2014; 73(12):2074–81.

12. Loricera J, Blanco R, Castañeda S, *et al*. Tocilizumab in refractory aortitis: study on 16 patients and literature review. *Clin Exp Rheumatol* 2014; 32(3 Suppl 82):S79–89.

13. Oliveira F, Butendieck RR, Ginsburg WW, *et al*. Tocilizumab, an effective treatment for relapsing giant cell arteritis. *Clin Exp Rheumatol* 2014; 32(3 Suppl 82):S76–8.

14. Al-Homood IA. Tocilizumab: a new therapy for large vessel vasculitis. *Clin Exp Med* 2014; 14(4):355–60.

15. Unizony SH, Dasgupta B, Fisheleva E, *et al*. Design of the tocilizumab in giant cell arteritis trial. *Int J Rheumatol* 2013; 2013:912562.

16. Ly K-H, Stirnemann J, Liozon E, *et al*. Interleukin-1 blockade in refractory giant cell arteritis. *Joint Bone Spine Rev Rhum* 2014; 81(1):76–8.

17. Volpe E, Servant N, Zollinger R, *et al*. A critical function for transforming growth factor-beta, interleukin 23 and proinflammatory cytokines in driving and modulating human T(H)-17 responses. *Nat Immunol* 2008; 9(6):650–7.

18. Matteson E, Dasgupta B, Schmidt W, *et al*. A 2-week single-blind, randomized, 3-arm proof of concept study of the effects of secukinumab (anti-IL17 mAb), canakinumab (anti-IL-1 b mAb), or corticosteroids on initial disease activity scores in patients with PMR, followed by an open-label extension to assess safety and effect duration. In *2014 ACR/ARHP Annual Meeting*, Boston, 2014. Abstract No 885. http://www.acrannualmeeting.org/wp-content/uploads/2014/10/2014-ACR_ARHP-Annual-Meeting-Program-Book-v2.pdf

19. Carruthers MN, Topazian MD, Khosroshahi A, *et al*. Rituximab for IgG4-related disease: a prospective, open-label trial. *Ann Rheum Dis* 2015; 74(6):1171–7.

20. Bhatia A, Ell PJ, Edwards JCW. Anti-CD20 monoclonal antibody (rituximab) as an adjunct in the treatment of giant cell arteritis. *Ann Rheum Dis* 2005; 64(7):1099–100.

21. Mayrbaeurl B, Hinterreiter M, Burgstaller S, *et al*. The first case of a patient with neutropenia and giant-cell arteritis treated with rituximab. *Clin Rheumatol* 2007; 26(9):1597–8.

22. Lozano E, Segarra M, García-Martínez A, *et al*. Imatinib mesylate inhibits in vitro and ex vivo biological responses related to vascular occlusion in giant cell arteritis. *Ann Rheum Dis* 2008; 67(11):1581–8.

Management of sight loss and other disease- and treatment-related complications

Pravin Patil, Niral Karia, and Bhaskar Dasgupta

> **Key points**
> - Sight loss and neuro-ophthalmic complications almost always arise prior to glucocorticoid therapy.
> - The commonest causes for sight loss are anterior ischaemic optic neuropathy and/or central retinal artery occlusion.
> - Sight loss in one eye predicts impending sight loss in the other eye.
> - Large-vessel vasculitis can have protean manifestations presenting as cranial and extracranial giant cell arteritis, refractory polymyalgic and constitutional symptoms, isolated aortitis, as well as a systemic syndrome.
> - Imaging has a critical role in elucidating disease extent in these situations.

103

13.1 Introduction

Acute sight loss secondary to ischaemic optic neuropathy or central retinal artery occlusion (Figure 13.1) is the most feared complication in giant cell arteritis (GCA) and can be considered as a 'stroke in the eye'. Sight loss can be a presenting symptom of GCA. Visual impairment may be preceded by diplopia, blurred vision, and transient loss, later becoming bilateral and irreversible if not treated immediately (Figure 13.2) (1). This has significant implications on personal, social care, and socioeconomic costs, along with an increased mortality within the first 5 years (2). It occurs in 20–50% of people with GCA if they are untreated (3).

13.2 Ophthalmic manifestations of giant cell arteritis

Acute visual loss in one or both eyes is by far the most feared and irreversible complication of GCA. The main blood supply compromised by GCA is to the anterior optic nerve head via the short posterior ciliary arteries and that of the retina via the central retinal artery. There is also choroidal ischaemia in GCA because short posterior ciliary arteries also supply this region.

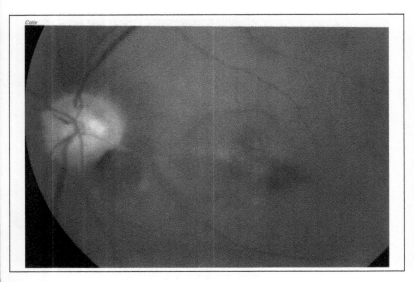

Figure 13.1 (See colour plate section). Central retinal occlusion in GCA.

In a Swiss study of 85 patients with GCA (including 78% biopsy-positive cases), the authors reported that 62 patients (73%) presented with ischaemic events which included jaw claudication, blurred vision, amaurosis fugax, permanent vision loss, and ischaemic stroke. In this study, 29 of 85 patients (34%) had permanent vision loss or stroke (4).

A retrospective Spanish study of 161 patients with biopsy-proven GCA found that 42 patients (26%) had visual manifestations of their disease, and of these patients, 24 (14.9%) developed permanent visual loss (9.9% unilateral, 5% bilateral) (5). Moreover, 7.5% of the patients experienced amaurosis fugax and 5.6% had diplopia before developing permanent loss of vision.

Permanent visual loss was caused by anterior ischaemic optic neuropathy in 91.7% and central retinal artery occlusion in 8.3%, and one patient had a vertebrobasilar stroke causing cortical visual loss.

An Italian study reported visual symptoms in 30.1% of their subjects, with partial or total visual loss in 19.1% (6). Of the 26 cases with visual loss, 92.3% were due to anterior ischaemic optic neuritis and 7.7% had central retinal artery occlusion. Visual loss was unilateral in 73.1% and bilateral in 26.9%. Furthermore, 25 of the 26 patients developed visual loss before corticosteroid therapy was started. However, visual manifestations may arise at any point in the natural course of the disease. If untreated, the other eye is likely to become affected within 1–2 weeks. Once established, visual impairment is usually permanent.

In a report by Ezeonyeji et al. of 65 patients with GCA, 23 patients had visual disturbance at presentation (35.3%) (7). Visual loss at presentation occurred in 16 patients (24.6%). Over 5 years, 19 patients were left with permanent visual impairment, eight of whom had bilateral loss of vision. Five patients had cerebrovascular complications, the majority of these being transient ischaemic attacks. One developed bilateral occipital infarcts with cortical blindness, and another developed oculomotor palsy. Ten patients (15.4%) presented with neuro-ophthalmic complications in the absence of headache, seven of whom (70%) developed permanent visual impairment. Five (7.7%)

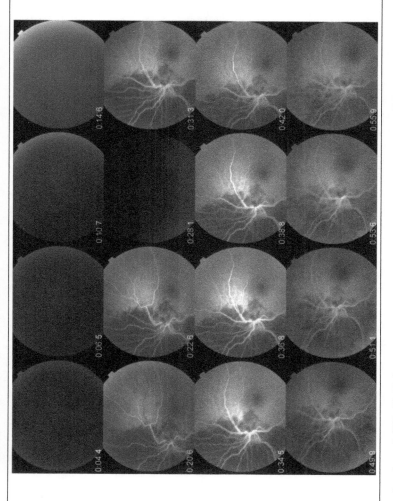

Figure 13.2 Fluorescein angiogram in GCA with sight loss.

patients had cerebrovascular complications. A significant minority of cases without headaches presented with constitutional, polymyalgic, and ischaemic symptoms.

13.3 Occult giant cell arteritis

Ophthalmology studies report occult GCA where visual loss is the presenting symptom. In a study of 85 patients, 21.2% of the patients with visual loss and positive temporal artery biopsy for GCA were reported not to have associated systemic symptoms (8). However, this may relate to lack of awareness of non-headache presentations such as constitutional and polymyalgic features leading to delayed diagnosis of GCA only after onset of permanent sight loss.

13.4 Predictors of visual loss and delayed recognition: 'symptom to steroid time'

Permanent visual loss is likely to occur in the very elderly, with a history of amaurosis fugax, jaw claudication, and temporal artery abnormalities on physical examination (9). Amaurosis fugax is an important visual symptom because it precedes permanent visual loss in 44% of patients. Delay in recognition may be the most important factor, given that the mean time from symptom onset to diagnosis of GCA was 35 days in the study by Ezeonyeji et al., and recognition of ischaemic symptoms was slow (7). Mackie et al. found that socioeconomic deprivation is associated with ischaemic complications (10), suggesting that lack of awareness and delay in recognition (particularly in the very elderly) may be contributory factors.

13.5 Diplopia

Transient or constant diplopia is a frequent visual symptom related to GCA. The reported incidence of diplopia in two large studies is approximately 6% (3, 5). Ophthalmoplegia in GCA is commonly associated with difficulty in upward gaze (11). Partial or complete IIIrd or VIth nerve palsy can be revealed on examination. The exact aetiology of ophthalmoplegia in GCA is not known. Ischaemia to the extraocular muscles, the cranial nerves, or brainstem ocular motor pathways have all been postulated as the mechanism of diplopia in GCA (12).

13.6 Unusual ocular manifestations

Rare ocular manifestations of GCA include tonic pupil (13), Horner syndrome (14), and internuclear ophthalmoplegia (15). Visual hallucinations seen in patients with cortical blindness are secondary to occipital infarction. Ocular ischaemic syndrome is another uncommon manifestation of GCA. It is a result of acute inflammatory thrombosis of multiple ciliary arteries causing ischaemia of both the anterior and posterior segment (16). The patients may be asymptomatic but have fundal blot haemorrhages with mild ocular hypotony.

13.7 Management of sight loss and the fast-track pathway

Sight loss in GCA almost always occurs prior to the institution of glucocorticoid (GC) therapy. A fast-track GCA pathway (Figure 13.3)—involving education and training of

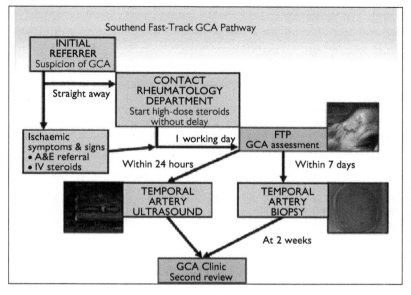

Figure 13.3 (See colour plate section). Southend Fast-Track GCA Pathway.

general practitioners and specialists, raising patient awareness, as well as rapid access clinics with facilities for vascular ultrasound and temporal artery biopsies reduces sight loss (17). This has also been found to be cost-effective. If there is no sight loss at the time of diagnosis and if treatment is instituted with high doses of GCs, the risk of sub-sequent sight loss is very small (18). Patients who already have some sight loss at the initial presentation, however, have a poorer prognosis and may even have increased mortality. One-quarter of patients develop further visual deterioration in the same eye, and up to 10% lose sight in the other eye, usually within the first few days (19). Patients with GCA-related sight loss may suffer loss of independence and residential home placement, severe depression, adverse effects from high-dose GCs, reduced quality-adjusted life years, and often injuries sustained (e.g. hip fractures) as a result of sight loss. In addition to these personal costs, there are also large healthcare and social costs related to blindness.

There are no trials comparing different GC dosing regimens in GCA. The recom-mendations are based on doses suggested in the British Society of Rheumatology (BSR) guidelines on GCA (Box 13.1).

Box 13.1 Treatment recommendations based on BSR guidelines

- Uncomplicated GCA (no jaw claudication or visual disturbance): 40–60 mg prednisolone daily
- Evolving visual loss (recent-onset visual symptoms over 6–12 hours or amaurosis fugax): intravenous methylprednisolone 500–1000 mg for 3 days before oral GCs
- Established visual loss: 60 mg prednisolone daily, to protect the contralateral eye.

13.8 Corticosteroid therapy

Early high-dose GC treatment is essential for rapid symptom control and to prevent further visual loss as far as possible (20). Most guidelines recommend oral prednisone 40–60 mg, once daily with consensus dictating higher doses in patients with ischaemic symptoms (21). In primary care practice, a dose of 60 mg daily should be used in most patients with suspected GCA and if necessary this can be adjusted once the patient has been assessed in secondary care.

Improvement in symptoms often begins within hours to days after commencing GCs, with a median time to initial response to an average initial dose of 60 mg/day being 8 days (22). Therefore, a lack of response is a strong indication that the initial diagnosis may have been incorrect (1).

Initial high-dose intravenous methylprednisolone is often used in clinical practice when patients present with threatened vision (20) although there is no evidence base, but this is the standard practice to avoid serious organ damage. It may also result in a reduction in cumulative steroid dosage after the use of intravenous GCs (23).

As a general guide, the BSR (21) suggests that the daily dose of prednisone is tapered as follows:

- Maintain the initial dose (40–60 mg) for at least 4 weeks, then
- Reduce by 10 mg, every 2 weeks, down to 20 mg, then
- Reduce by 2.5 mg, every 2–4 weeks, to 10 mg, then
- Reduce by 1 mg, every 4–8 weeks, provided there are no relapses.

13.9 Additional treatment

Daily aspirin may be considered for patients without contraindications as there is some evidence that it decreases the rate of visual loss and other cerebrovascular complications (21). Use of low-dose aspirin should be counterbalanced against the risk of gastrointestinal bleeding, especially with co-prescription of GCs.

The key learning points on this topic are summarized in Box 13.2.

13.10 Complications of giant cell arteritis

GCA is too often considered as a disease of the temporal arteries only. It is important that the concept of a headache-dominated cranial GCA picture is broadened to include the 'vascular' view of GCA. This takes into account other significant problems that can occur in GCA patients. Severe cases of GCA may lead to numbness or infarction of the scalp (Figure 13.4) or the tongue. It is now well established that GCA patients should

---

Box 13.2 Learning points on giant cell arteritis

- Acute irreversible visual loss in one or both eyes is the most feared complication of GCA and almost always occurs before GC therapy.
- Delay in recognition of GCA is an important factor for GCA-related visual impairment.
- Where there is a strong clinical suspicion of GCA, a delay in treatment will almost always have greater consequences than an unnecessary dose of GCs in someone who is later found to not have the condition.

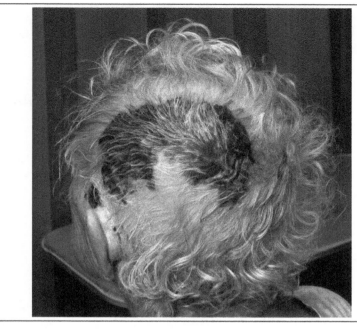

Figure 13.4 (See colour plate section). Scalp necrosis in GCA.

be actively screened for extracranial disease, particularly given the fact that this is often clinically silent. If undetected, extracranial large-vessel vasculitis (LVV) (Figure 13.5) can result in serious sequelae such as stroke and aortic aneurysm (Figure 13.6). Large-vessel stenosis, and with it an increased risk of stroke, occurs in 10–15% of people (24).

The mortality rate in GCA patients is not significantly different from the general population (25). However, the risk of aortic aneurysm is reported to be 17 times greater in

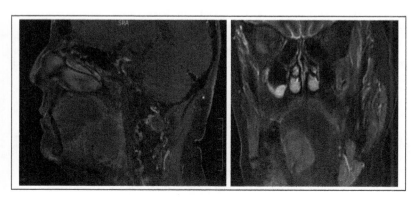

Figure 13.5 Other serious pathology mimicking GCA.

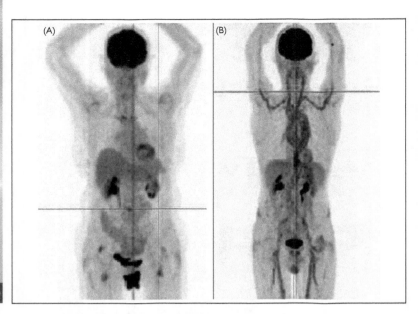

Figure 13.6 ^{18}F-FDG-PET scans of two GCA patients with suspected extracranial involvement. (A) No elevated ^{18}F-FDG uptake in the large vessels. (B) Pathologically elevated ^{18}F-FDG uptake in the aorta and its major branches seen in a 69-year-old GCA patient with polymyalgia and profound constitutional symptoms.

people who have had GCA, when compared to the general population of the same age and sex (25). Findings on fluorine-18-labelled fluorodeoxyglucose-positron emission tomography with computed tomography (FDG-PET/CT) scanning and arterial ultrasound suggest that subclinical involvement of the large vessels is common, a major clinical consequence of which is aortic aneurysm, described in 10–18% of reported series (26, 27). Arterial involvement in GCA is not limited only to the thoracic or abdominal aorta. Upper and/or lower limb inflammatory arteritis during GCA is not exceptional occurring in 3–16% of patients (28). It is rarely reported in the literature but is probably underestimated as it is often asymptomatic.

Annual monitoring with chest X-ray and ultrasound, and the management of modifiable risk factors, such as hypertension, smoking, and central obesity, may help to reduce this risk. Clinical awareness should be maintained during the follow-up period as aneurysms may not manifest for several years after the initial diagnosis of GCA. Patients should have a chest radiograph every 2 years to monitor for aortic aneurysm. In suspected large-vessel GCA, this may need supplementation with echocardiography,

---

Box 13.3 Learning points on complications of giant cell arteritis

- Late diagnosis of extracranial LVV in GCA patients may lead to serious complications such as stroke and aortic aneurysm.
- In suspected extracranial LVV patients, imaging with FDG-PET should be considered (Figure 13.7).

FDG-PET/CT, magnetic resonance imaging/CT as appropriate (21). FDG-PET/CT is well suited to the assessment of activity and extent of large vessel vasculitis.

There are several unanswered questions regarding aneurysms in GCA. It is neither possible to predict who will go on to develop aneurysms nor it is clear whether aggressive treatment reduces the risk of developing aneurysms. In addition, the cost-effectiveness of screening has not yet been carried out.

The key points on this topic can be found in Box 13.3.

13.11 Complications of polymyalgia rheumatica

As polymyalgia rheumatica (PMR) can have a non-specific clinical presentation (see Chapter 9), it should be diagnosed with caution. A history and clinical examination including an assessment for symptoms and signs of GCA, such as scalp tenderness, temporal artery tenderness, and new-onset or new type of headache, should be included in each follow-up. If symptoms of GCA arise, the patient should be presumed to have the condition (29). Also, assess for symptoms and signs of adverse effects of GCs.

Patients with PMR have a higher likelihood of having a history of myocardial infarction (odds ratio (OR) 1.78; 95% confidence interval (CI) 1.13–2.82), peripheral vascular diseases (OR 2.21; 95% CI: 1.37–3.60), and cerebrovascular diseases (OR 1.60; 95% CI 1.08–2.39) (30). These comorbidities increase costs (e.g. for hospital stays and imaging) compared to matched non-PMR subjects (30). Management of comorbidities including cardiovascular risks such as hypertension, diabetes, hyperlipidaemia, obesity, and osteoporosis is necessary throughout the entire course of the disease.

Vascular involvement in PMR is increasingly recognized though imaging modalities addressed elsewhere in this book. These studies strengthen the suggestion of a vasculitic nature to many cases of PMR (polymyalgia arteritica). The long-term vascular damage due to such vascular inflammation is unknown. However, there are reports of subsequent aortic dilatation in patients with aortic involvement on FDG-PET/CT scanning.

FDG-PET/CT scan should be considered in a subgroup of PMR-resistant or partially responsive to GCs patients. GC resistance means inability to taper prednisolone dose to less than 7.5 mg daily without exacerbations (31). These patients may benefit from addition of an adjuvant agent such as leflunomide (32).

13.12 Strategies for detection and management of adverse effects

GCs are the mainstay of treatment in both PMR and GCA. A treatment course of 2–3 years is often necessary, with some patients requiring low-dose prednisone for several years thereafter. GC-related adverse effects are therefore common, occurring in approximately 60% of patients (22). This is worsened by the fact that a significant number of patients have pre-existing comorbidities such as diabetes mellitus, hypertension, and heart disease. Hence, risk stratification of therapy, as stressed by the European League Against Rheumatism/American College of Rheumatology PMR guidelines, based on demographics, co-morbidities, disease severity and damage, as well as patient preferences is the way forward (33).

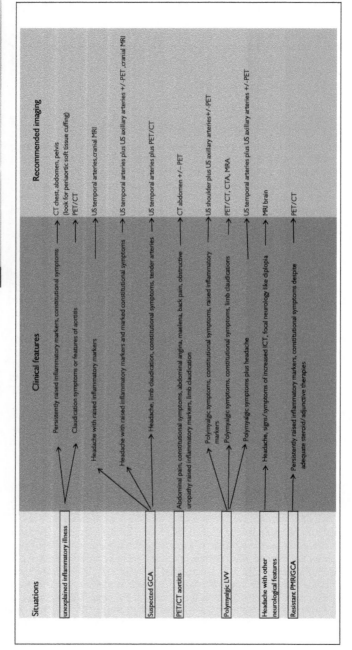

Figure 13.7 Imaging in patients with suspected LVV.

> Box 13.4 Common adverse effects of corticosteroids
>
> - Skin changes and disorders (e.g. thinning and bruising, striae, acne, alopecia, and hirsutism)
> - Body composition changes (e.g. weight gain, Cushingoid features)
> - Ocular disorders (e.g. glaucoma and cataracts)
> - Gastrointestinal disorders (e.g. dyspepsia, oesophagitis, gastritis, ulcers, and bleeding)
> - Central nervous system changes (e.g. sleep disturbance, mood changes, restlessness, depression, and psychosis)
> - Renal changes (e.g. hypertension and fluid retention)
> - Diabetes
> - Osteoporosis.

13.12.1 Adverse effects of corticosteroids

Major risks associated with GCs include the development of diabetes mellitus and osteoporotic fractures. Box 13.4 lists some of the important complications of GCs. Older age, higher cumulative doses of GCs, and female sex increase the risk of occurrence of adverse effects (22). To minimize the risk, practice points mentioned in Box 13.5 should be implemented.

13.12.1.1 *Osteoporosis prophylaxis*

Rapid bone loss and increased fracture risk occur soon after the initiation of GC therapy. Fracture risk is dependent on dose and treatment duration. Ideally a bone mineral density scan of the lumbar spine and hip should be requested for patients when starting long-term GCs; however, this depends on the availability and funding of the local service.

The American College of Rheumatology 2010 and UK National Institute for Health and Care Excellence guidance for osteoporosis recommendations underline that vitamin D supplements should be given. Adequate dietary calcium, or supplementation if this is not possible, is also necessary.

> Box 13.5 Practice points to consider whenever a patient is prescribed glucocorticoids long term
>
> - The patient's co-morbidities and risk factors for adverse effects should be evaluated and managed. These include hypertension, diabetes, peptic ulcer, recent fractures, cataract/glaucoma, chronic infection, dyslipidaemia, and concurrent non-steroidal anti-inflammatory drug (NSAID) use.
> - During the course of treatment, monitor body weight and blood pressure, and assess for peripheral oedema and heart failure.
> - Consider testing for serum lipids, HbA_{1c} (or fasting glucose in the first 2 months) depending on the individual patient's risk of adverse effects, dose, and duration.
> - Patients who experience adverse gastrointestinal affects or taking NSAIDS with GCs should be given appropriate gastroprotective medicines.
> - Patients taking GC treatment for longer than 1 month, who need to undergo surgery, will require perioperative management with adequate GC replacement to overcome potential adrenal insufficiency.
> - Tapering must be done carefully to avoid relapses of the condition and potential adrenal deficiency.

Bisphosphonates are the front-line choice for prevention of fracture. Fracture risk can be assessed using the FRAX® algorithm, although risk may be underestimated in patients taking higher doses of GCs. All patients with GCA should be initially co-prescribed bisphosphonates. In PMR, addition of bisphosphonate is required in the following high-risk patients for major osteoporotic fractures (34):

* Postmenopausal women
* Men aged 50 years or older
* T-score is −1.5 or lower
* History of fragility fractures.

The issue of toxicities due to GCs has prompted the search for other therapies for GCA, especially those with steroid-sparing qualities. The proven ability of timely administration of GCs to prevent blindness in GCA is a yardstick against which any other treatment must be measured. While awaiting development of safer therapies we could concentrate efforts in reducing 'symptom-to-steroid' time. A fast-track pathway for management of GCA is one such example (17).

13.13 **Conclusion**

Despite the issues surrounding the management of GCA, we do have a dramatically effective treatment for the prevention of blindness in GCA: the fast-track GCA pathway and the expeditious use of higher doses of GCs. Patients should be informed of the adverse effects associated with GCs and may need to be advised to make lifestyle changes to lower their risk of complications. The chronic complications of PMR and GCA often go unrecognized. Newer imaging modalities hold promise for better assessment. While awaiting better ways of managing GCA and PMR we must continue to share knowledge with colleagues in other disciplines about these common systemic rheumatic diseases, so that patients may reap benefits of timely diagnosis and appropriate treatment.

References

1. Dasgupta B. Concise guidance: diagnosis and management of giant cell arteritis. *Clin Med* 2010; 10(4):381–6.

2. Crow RW, Katz BJ, Warner JE, et al. Giant cell arteritis and mortality. *J Gerontol A Biol Sci Med Sci* 2009; 64(3):365–9.

3. Hayreh SS, Podhajsky PA, Zimmerman B. Ocular manifestations of giant cell arteritis. *Am J Ophthalmol* 1998; 125(4):509–20.

4. Berger CT, Wolbers M, Meyer P, et al. High incidence of severe ischaemic complications in patients with giant cell arteritis irrespective of platelet count and size, and platelet inhibition. *Rheumatology (Oxford)* 2009; 48(3):258–61.

5. González-Gay MA, García-Porrúa C, Llorca J, et al. Visual manifestations of giant cell arteritis. Trends and clinical spectrum in 161 patients. *Medicine (Baltimore)* 2000; 79(5):283–92.

6. Salvarani C, Cimino L, Macchioni P, et al. Risk factors for visual loss in an Italian population-based cohort of patients with giant cell arteritis. *Arthritis Rheum* 2005; 53(2):293–7.

7. Ezeonyeji AN, Borg FA, Dasgupta B. Delays in recognition and management of giant cell arteritis: results from a retrospective audit. *Clin Rheumatol* 2011; 30(2):259–62.

8. Hayreh SS, Podhajsky PA, Zimmerman B. Occult giant cell arteritis: ocular manifestations. *Am J Ophthalmol* 1998; 125(4):521–6.

9. Borg FA, Salter VLJ, Dasgupta B. Neuro-ophthalmic complications in giant cell arteritis. *Curr Allergy Asthma Rep* 2008; 8(4):323–30.

10. Mackie SL, Dasgupta B, Hordon L, *et al*. Ischaemic manifestations in giant cell arteritis are associated with area level socio-economic deprivation, but not cardiovascular risk factors. *Rheumatology (Oxford)* 2011; 50(11):2014–22.

11. Reich K, Giansiracusa D, Strongwater S. Neurologic manifestations of giant cell arteritis. *Am J Med* 1996; 89(1):67–72.

12. Kawasaki A, Purvin V. Giant cell arteritis: an updated review. *Acta Ophthalmol* 2009; 87(1):13–32.

13. Foroozan R, Buono LM, Savino P, *et al*. Tonic pupils from giant cell arteritis. *Br J Opthalmol* 2003; 87(4):500–19.

14. Shah A V, Paul-Oddoye AB, Madill SA, *et al*. Horner's syndrome associated with giant cell arteritis. *Eye (Lond)* 2007; 21(1):130–1.

15. Ahmad I, Zaman M. Bilateral internuclear ophthalmoplegia: an initial presenting sign of giant cell arteritis. *J Am Geriatr Soc* 1999; 47(6):734–6.

16. Mendrinos E, Machinis TG, Pournaras CJ. Ocular ischemic syndrome. *Surv Ophthalmol* 2010; 55(1):2–34.

17. Patil P, Williams M, Maw WW, *et al*. Fast track pathway reduces sight loss in giant cell arteritis: results of a longitudinal observational cohort study. *Clin Exp Rheumatol* 2015; 33(2 Suppl 89):103–6.

18. Aiello PD, Trautmann JC, McPhee TJ, *et al*. Visual prognosis in giant cell arteritis. *Ophthalmology* 1993; 100(4):550–5.

19. Danesh-Meyer H, Savino PJ, Gamble GG. Poor prognosis of visual outcome after visual loss from giant cell arteritis. *Ophthalmology* 2005; 112(6):1098–103.

20. Hayreh SS, Zimmerman B. Visual deterioration in giant cell arteritis patients while on high doses of corticosteroid therapy. *Ophthalmology* 2003; 110(6):1204–15.

21. Dasgupta B, Borg FA, Hassan N, *et al*. BSR and BHPR guidelines for the management of giant cell arteritis. *Rheumatology (Oxford)* 2010; 49(8):1594–7.

22. Proven A, Gabriel SE, Orces C, *et al*. Glucocorticoid therapy in giant cell arteritis: duration and adverse outcomes. *Arthritis Rheum* 2003; 49(5):703–8.

23. Mazlumzadeh M, Hunder GG, Easley KA, *et al*. Treatment of giant cell arteritis using induction therapy with high-dose glucocorticoids: a double-blind, placebo-controlled, randomized prospective clinical trial. *Arthritis Rheum* 2006; 54(10):3310–18.

24. Kermani TA, Warrington KJ, Crowson CS, *et al*. Large-vessel involvement in giant cell arteritis: a population-based cohort study of the incidence-trends and prognosis. *Ann Rheum Dis* 2013; 72(12):1989–94.

25. BMJ Best Practice. *Giant Cell Arteritis* [Online]. 2013. http://bestpractice.bmj.com/best-practice/monograph/177.html

26. Blockmans D, de Ceuninck L, Vanderschueren S, *et al*. Repetitive 18F-fluorodeoxyglucose positron emission tomography in giant cell arteritis: a prospective study of 35 patients. *Arthritis Rheum* 2006; 55(1):131–7.

27. Schmidt WA, Seifert A, Gromnica-Ihle E, *et al*. Ultrasound of proximal upper extremity arteries to increase the diagnostic yield in large-vessel giant cell arteritis. *Rheumatology (Oxford)* 2008; 47(1):96–101.

28. Daumas A, Bernard F, Rossi P, *et al*. "Extra-cranial" manifestations of giant cell arteritis. In Amezcua-Guerra LM (ed) *Advances in the Diagnosis and Treatment of Vasculitis*. Rijeka, Croatia: InTech, 2011:291–310.

29. Dasgupta B, Borg F, Hassan N, *et al*. BSR and BHPR guidelines for the management of polymyalgia rheumatica. *Rheumatology (Oxford)* 2010; 49(1):186–90.

30. Kremers HM, Reinalda MS, Crowson CS, *et al*. Direct medical costs of polymyalgia rheumatica. *Arthritis Rheum* 2005; 53(4):578–84.

31. Cimmino M, Zampogna G, Parodi M. Is FDG-PET useful in the evaluation of steroid-resistant PMR patients? *Rheumatology (Oxford)* 2008; 47(6):926–7.

32. Adizie T, Christidis D, Dharmapaliah C, *et al*. Efficacy and tolerability of leflunomide in difficult-to-treat polymyalgia rheumatica and giant cell arteritis: a case series. *Int J Clin Pract* 2012; 66(9):906–9.

33. Dejaco C, Singh YP, Perel P, *et al*. 2015 Recommendations for the management of polymyalgia rheumatica: a European League Against Rheumatism/American College of Rheumatology collaborative initiative. *Ann Rheum Dis* 2015; 74(10):1799–807.

34. Grossman JM, Gordon R, Ranganath VK, *et al*. American College of Rheumatology 2010 recommendations for the prevention and treatment of glucocorticoid-induced osteoporosis. *Arthritis Care Res (Hoboken)* 2010; 62(11):1515–26.

Part 4

Outcomes, prognosis, socioeconomic implications, primary care, and patient perspectives

14 Determination of disease activity and outcomes   119

15 Prognosis and duration of therapy   125

16 Primary care   133

17 Socioeconomic implications   139

18 Patient education   145

Chapter 14

Determination of disease activity and outcomes

Christian Dejaco

Key points

- Clinical criteria for assessment of disease activity in polymyalgia rheumatica (PMR) and giant cell arteritis (GCA) have not been established so far.
- Elevation of inflammatory markers in the absence of other signs of disease activity is not sufficient to justify a change of treatment.
- The role of imaging methods for the assessment of disease activity in PMR and GCA is unclear. Ultrasound, magnetic resonance imaging, and fluorodeoxyglucose-positron emission tomography may be used to monitor active vasculitis of large vessels and the aorta.

14.1 Introduction

Criteria for the assessment of disease activity in PMR and GCA have not been established so far. In clinical studies and routine practice, symptoms and laboratory parameters are commonly used to determine current disease state; however, these factors generally lack sensitivity and specificity. In addition, pain symptoms are often difficult to interpret given that elderly patients frequently suffer from comorbidities that may cause similar complaints to PMR and/or GCA (1). Recent studies suggest that imaging techniques such as ultrasound, magnetic resonance imaging (MRI), and/or fluorine-18-labelled fluorodeoxyglucose-positron emission tomography (^{18}F-FDG-PET) may support objective assessment of disease activity in PMR and GCA (2, 3). The PMR activity score (PMR-AS), a composite score for PMR, has been proposed for measurement of disease activity in clinical practice and trials; however, this score is still infrequently used and requires further validation (4).

14.2 Determination of disease activity

14.2.1 Remission and relapse criteria in polymyalgia rheumatica

'Remission' is the most common therapeutic goal of PMR patients because of the rapid and complete response of symptoms after initiation of glucocorticoid (GC) treatment (1).

Box 14.1 Parameters for assessment of remission and relapse in polymyalgia rheumatica agreed upon in an international consensus project

- Morning stiffness
- Erythrocyte sedimentation rate
- C-reactive protein
- Patient's assessment of pain related to neck, upper arms, shoulders, and pelvic girdle (VAS)
- Corticosteroid dose required to control symptoms
- Shoulder-pain worsened by passive and active mobilization
- Limitation of upper limb elevation
- Clinical signs of coxo-femoral synovitis.[a]

VAS, visual analogue scale with 0 = no pain, 10 = unbearable pain on a 10 cm scale.

[a] Coxo-femoral synovitis is suggested if the patient complains about pain in the groin worsened by passive and active movements on clinical examination.

Source data from Leeb BF, Bird HA. A disease activity score for polymyalgia rheumatica. *Ann Rheum Dis* 2004; 63:1279–83.

A relapse of the disease prompts physicians to change current therapy, in most cases by an increment of the GC dose (5). For both clinical states, various definitions have been used in the literature and it is still a matter of discussion whether a definition is required for either state, or whether a relapse is simply the absence of remission (1).

The parameters most commonly used in the literature to define remission are the absence of clinical signs of PMR (pain and stiffness) plus normalized acute phase reactants. An isolated raise of the erythrocyte sedimentation rate (ESR) or C-reactive protein (CRP) without a worsening of PMR symptoms is usually not sufficient to diagnose a relapse whereas a worsening of shoulder and/or hip pain without an elevation of acute phase reactants may be caused by other painful conditions such as concomitant osteoarthritis or degenerative disease of the rotator cuff. The combination of clinical and laboratory criteria as just described is thus the most specific method for remission and relapse assessment in PMR. No data from prospective studies, however, exist about the value of individual clinical (e.g. shoulder pain, hip pain, and elevation of upper limb) and laboratory parameters. Moreover, optimal cut-offs for these parameters that reliably distinguish active from inactive disease are so far elusive (5–7). A Delphi exercise has recently been conducted among international experts of PMR and GCA to agree upon a set of parameters that may be used to define remission and relapse in PMR (1). The items resulting from this study are listed in Box 14.1. Prospective studies are now required to evaluate the relevance of these factors.

14.2.2 Polymyalgia rheumatica activity score

The PMR-AS is the only composite index for PMR available, combining CRP (alternatively ESR), pain and global disease activity assessment by the patient and the physician, respectively, duration of morning stiffness, and the ability to elevate the arms (see Box 14.2 for details) (4, 8). Cut-offs defining states of remission, low, moderate, and high disease activity as well as relapse have been proposed (Box 14.2); however, the value of these definitions still has to be clarified (4, 8–10).

14.2.3 Disease activity measurement in giant cell arteritis

Clinical criteria determining disease activity in GCA are not yet available (6, 11). A worsening of GCA characteristic symptoms (such as headache or visual symptoms)

Box 14.2 Calculation of the PMR-AS and suggested cut-offs for different disease activity states

---

PMR-AS = CRP (mg/dL) + patient's pain assessment (VAS 0–10)[a] + physician's global assessment (VAS 0–10)[b] + (morning stiffness (minutes) × 0.1) + EUL (0–3)[c]

- Remission: 0–1.5
- Low disease activity: 1.6–6.9
- Moderate disease activity: 7.0–17.0
- High disease activity: > 17.0
- Relapse: > 9.35 or a ΔPMR-AS score > 6.6

CRP, C-reactive protein; EUL, ability to elevate the upper limbs; VAS, visual analogue scale.

[a] 0 = no pain, 10 = unbearable pain; [b] 0 = no disease activity, 10 = activity highest possible; [c] 0 = above shoulder girdle, 1 = up to shoulder girdle; 2 = below shoulder girdle; 3 = none.

---

and/or abnormal results of clinical examination of temporal and/or extracranial arteries such as tenderness, swelling, new bruits, and so on, in conjunction with an increment of inflammatory markers suggest a relapse (12). Similar to current clinical practice in PMR, an isolated rise of ESR or CRP in GCA patients does not justify a change of therapy and normal acute phase reactants in symptomatic GCA patients should tempt suspicion of an alternative diagnosis (6).

The most sensitive laboratory parameters for a flare of GCA are CRP and interleukin (IL)-6 whereas ESR is less useful for relapse diagnosis (13). The IL-6 assay, however, is not routinely available in most non-academic hospitals and private practice and given that IL-6 and CRP levels correlate well, the assessment of IL-6 may be dispensable for routine assessment of disease activity in GCA (14).

14.3 **Imaging methods for determination of disease activity**

Ultrasound, MRI, and ^{18}F-FDG-PET have been studied as possible markers of disease activity in PMR and GCA. In PMR, ultrasound and ^{18}F-FDG-PET studies demonstrated a reduction of inflammatory changes at joints and bursae along with clinical improvement and normalization of acute phase reactants during follow-up (15–17). In a proportion of patients, however, imaging-detected inflammation persisted despite clinical remission. The relevance of these findings is still unclear given that the presence of subclinical inflammation was not associated with a higher short-term relapse rate (17).

In GCA, ultrasound has been used in patients with temporal arteritis as well as in cases with extracranial large-vessel vasculitis in order to monitor the disappearance of the 'halo' sign in patients responding to GC treatment (18, 19). The significance of a persisting 'halo' despite clinical improvement as well as the recurrence of a 'halo' sign in patients without a clinical relapse of GCA is unknown (20). In the long-term follow-up of GCA patients, ultrasound of the abdominal aorta may be valuable to identify patients developing an aortic aneurysm (6). A specific recommendation about whether any, all, or a subpopulation of GCA patients (e.g. those with risk factors for aneurysm development such as patients with male sex, smoking history, hypertension, or inflammatory uptake of the aorta at baseline as assessed by ^{18}F-FDG-PET) should be regularly screened by abdominal ultrasound scans (and at which intervals) cannot be given at this stage (21, 22).

MRI and ^{18}F-FDG-PET of large vessels are often used to monitor disease activity in GCA patients with inflammation of extracranial large vessels and/or the aorta, particularly in cases with mild or unspecific symptoms plus raised acute phase reactants (6). In patients with cranial symptoms, high-resolution MRI may also be valuable to detect inflammation of cranial arteries (23, 24). The specificity of ^{18}F-FDG-PET and MRI findings, however, is still a matter of debate given that inflammatory changes may be found in a considerable proportion of GCA patients in clinical remission and conversely, seemingly unaffected vessels may develop inflammatory damage lesions later during follow-up (24).

14.4 Outcomes relevant to polymyalgia rheumatica and giant cell arteritis

The relief of symptoms and the prevention of disease-specific complications (e.g. progression of PMR to GCA, vascular occlusion/stenosis, and/or aortic aneurysms in GCA) while minimizing the risk of treatment-related toxicity is the desired short-term treatment outcome of PMR and GCA by most physicians. 'Being on steroids' and 'living with steroids' are among the most important concepts to patients according to a survey conducted by PMRGCAuk (25). Indeed, more than 50% of PMR and GCA patients suffer from at least one GC-related adverse event and the reduction of the cumulative GC dose has been one of the most important goals of clinical studies of immunosuppressive agents.

Patient-reported outcome parameters specifically developed and evaluated for PMR and GCA are not yet available. A recent prospective study in PMR identified pain, loss of function, morning stiffness, and mental impairment (as measured by Short Form-36 questionnaire) as possible items for a patient-reported outcome measurement tool (26). Further research including studies using a qualitative approach is required in this field.

References

1. Dejaco C, Duftner C, Cimmino MA, et al. Definition of remission and relapse in polymyalgia rheumatica: data from a literature search compared with a Delphi-based expert consensus. Ann Rheum Dis 2011; 70:447–53.

2. Camellino D, Cimmino MA. Imaging of polymyalgia rheumatica: indications on its pathogenesis, diagnosis and prognosis. Rheumatology (Oxford) 2012; 51:77–86.

3. Dejaco C, Schirmer M, Duftner C. [Expectations of rheumatologists on imaging results]. Radiologe 2012; 52:110–15.

4. Leeb BF, Bird HA. A disease activity score for polymyalgia rheumatica. Ann Rheum Dis 2004; 63:1279–83.

5. Duftner C, Dejaco C, Schirmer M. [Polymyalgia rheumatica]. Internist (Berl) 2009; 50:51–7.

6. Dejaco C, Duftner C, Dasgupta B, et al. Polymyalgia rheumatica and giant cell arteritis: management of two diseases of the elderly. Aging Health 2011; 7:633–45.

7. Dasgupta B, Borg FA, Hassan N, et al. BSR and BHPR guidelines for the management of polymyalgia rheumatica. Rheumatology (Oxford) 2010; 49:186–90.

8. Leeb BF, Bird HA, Nesher G, et al. EULAR response criteria for polymyalgia rheumatica: results of an initiative of the European Collaborating Polymyalgia Rheumatica Group (subcommittee of ESCISIT). Ann Rheum Dis 2003; 62:1189–94.

9. Leeb BF, Rintelen B, Sautner J, et al. The polymyalgia rheumatica activity score in daily use: proposal for a definition of remission. *Arthritis Rheum* 2007; 57:810–15.

10. Binard A, de Bandt M, Berthelot JM, et al. Performance of the polymyalgia rheumatica activity score for diagnosing disease flares. *Arthritis Rheum* 2008; 59:263–9.

11. Mukhtyar C, Guillevin L, Cid MC, et al. EULAR recommendations for the management of large vessel vasculitis. *Ann Rheum Dis* 2009; 68:318–23.

12. Dejaco C, Wipfler-Freißmuth E, Duftner C, et al. Assessment of disease activity of systemic vasculitides in clinical practice. *Aktuel Rheumatol* 2009; 34:180–5.

13. Salvarani C, Cantini F, Niccoli L, et al. Acute-phase reactants and the risk of relapse/recurrence in polymyalgia rheumatica: a prospective followup study. *Arthritis Rheum* 2005; 53:33–8.

14. Salvarani C, Cantini F, Boiardi L, et al. Laboratory investigations useful in giant cell arteritis and Takayasu's arteritis. *Clin Exp Rheumatol* 2003; 21:S23–8.

15. Blockmans D, De Ceuninck L, Vanderschueren S, et al. Repetitive 18-fluorodeoxyglucose positron emission tomography in isolated polymyalgia rheumatica: a prospective study in 35 patients. *Rheumatology (Oxford)* 2007; 46:672–7.

16. Jimenez-Palop M, Naredo E, Humbrado L, et al. Ultrasonographic monitoring of response to therapy in polymyalgia rheumatica. *Ann Rheum Dis* 2010; 69:879–82.

17. Macchioni P, Catanoso MG, Pipitone N, et al. Longitudinal examination with shoulder ultrasound of patients with polymyalgia rheumatica. *Rheumatology (Oxford)* 2009; 48:1566–9.

18. Besada E, Nossent JC. Ultrasonographic resolution of the vessel wall oedema with modest clinical improvement in a large-vessel vasculitis patient treated with tocilizumab. *Clin Rheumatol* 2012; 31:1263–5.

19. Pipitone N, Versari A, Salvarani C. Role of imaging studies in the diagnosis and follow-up of large-vessel vasculitis: an update. *Rheumatology (Oxford)* 2008; 47:403–8.

20. Aschwanden M, Kesten F, Stern M, et al. Vascular involvement in patients with giant cell arteritis determined by duplex sonography of 2x11 arterial regions. *Ann Rheum Dis* 2010; 69:1356–9.

21. Robson JC, Kiran A, Maskell J, et al. The relative risk of aortic aneurysm in patients with giant cell arteritis compared with the general population of the UK. *Ann Rheum Dis* 2015; 74:129–35.

22. Blockmans D, Coudyzer W, Vanderschueren S, et al. Relationship between fluorodeoxyglucose uptake in the large vessels and late aortic diameter in giant cell arteritis. *Rheumatology (Oxford)* 2008; 47:1179–84.

23. Bley TA, Uhl M, Venhoff N, et al. 3-T MRI reveals cranial and thoracic inflammatory changes in giant cell arteritis. *Clin Rheumatol* 2007; 26:448–50.

24. Blockmans D, Bley T, Schmidt W. Imaging for large-vessel vasculitis. *Curr Opin Rheumatol* 2009; 21:19–28.

25. Gilbert K. *Polymyalgia Rheumatica and Giant Cell Arteritis: A Survival Guide.* London: PMRGCAuk, 2014.

26. Matteson EL, Maradit-Kremers H, Cimmino MA, et al. Patient-reported outcomes in polymyalgia rheumatica. *J Rheumatol* 2012; 39:795–803.

Chapter 15

Prognosis and duration of therapy

Sarah L. Mackie

Key points

- Patients with polymyalgia rheumatica (PMR) may be diagnosed with giant cell arteritis (GCA) before, at the same time, or after diagnosis of PMR.
- The risk of developing irreversible, ischaemic complications (such as blindness or stroke) is minimized by means of good patient education about warning signs to watch out for and early diagnosis.
- Some patients with GCA (especially imaging-proven large-vessel GCA) develop aortic complications, including aneurysm, dissection, or rupture, some years later.
- Patients with both PMR and GCA are usually treated with glucocorticoids for longer than those with isolated PMR.
- To avoid relapses, PMR and GCA both usually require 1–2 years of systemic glucocorticoid therapy, gradually tapered before finally stopping.
- The duration of glucocorticoid therapy depends on the rate of tapering of glucocorticoids, which should be a decision made between physician and patient on an individual basis.
- Patients with PMR or GCA who are female, or who have higher inflammatory markers before treatment, usually receive glucocorticoids for a longer duration.
- Measures should be taken to reduce any modifiable risks relating to drug-related complications, particularly those relating to glucocorticoids.

125

15.1 Prognosis: general considerations

15.1.1 Patient selection

Published data on the prognosis of PMR and GCA reflect the way that patients were selected (Box 15.1). Single-speciality studies can introduce bias, for example, due to differences between the 'cranial' and 'large-vessel' variants of GCA (1, 2); these different phenotypic expressions of disease are often differentially represented in different specialities (e.g. ophthalmology, rheumatology, acute medicine, and geriatrics). Technologies such as biopsy and imaging used to identify patients may also introduce bias.

- Evaluate for symptoms and signs of PMR and GCA and adjust glucocorticoid dose accordingly
- If new GCA suspected—act urgently
- Blood pressure (consider checking both arms)
- Falls, skin fragility, and fracture risk assessment
- Diabetes assessment
- Discuss continuation of valued activities including physical activity
- Assessment of potential impact of glucocorticoids on coexisting medical conditions
- Tell the patient about the features of GCA to watch out for, and what to do if they occur
- Review 'steroid card' (and remind patient about what to do in the event of inter-current illness or surgery, if iatrogenic adrenal insufficiency is a possibility)
- Signpost to peer and other support networks as appropriate.

15.1.2 **Polymyalgia rheumatica and giant cell arteritis**

Apparently isolated PMR can show imaging or biopsy features of GCA (3). Leaving aside the question of whether or not they are the same disease, PMR and GCA coexist frequently in clinical practice: if the patient has one of these diseases, they are at elevated risk of developing the other disease at a later date.

15.1.3 **Case ascertainment**

Methods of case ascertainment in GCA may introduce bias. Since the 1990 American College of Rheumatology classification criteria for GCA are somewhat over-inclusive for clinical practice (4), inclusion of cases in GCA cohorts may require more stringent criteria, such as a positive temporal artery biopsy. But not all patients with GCA have a positive biopsy. Large-vessel vasculitis (LVV) that affects the aorta and its proximal branches, but may spare the temporal artery (1), may also have fewer cranial manifestations than biopsy-proven GCA (2).

For PMR, confirmation of diagnosis always requires clinical expertise, and this presents a problem for case ascertainment in prognostic studies. Studies with longitudinal follow-up are usually able to exclude patients who later received an alternative explanation for their PMR-like symptoms (a change in diagnosis), such as infection, cancer, or inflammatory arthritis (5). This 'polymyalgic-onset rheumatoid arthritis' is well recognized, but is probably most common within rheumatology clinics, where there is greater readiness to consider adjuvant immunosuppressant therapy (6).

15.1.4 **Treatment goals and relapses**

Tapering of glucocorticoid therapy should be individualized based on individual patient factors, including the estimated risk of glucocorticoid-related adverse effects, co-morbidities, and patient preference. Principles of treatment include minimizing cumulative glucocorticoid exposure whilst maintaining sustained disease control in order to reduce the risk of relapse. Definitions of relapse vary in different studies, probably reflecting different treatment approaches as well as the study goal.

15.2 Irreversible cranial ischaemic complications

Once treatment has been established, irreversible ischaemic complications such as blindness or stroke are very uncommon after the first 2 weeks of treatment (7, 8). Patients with PMR and GCA are educated about which ischaemic symptoms of GCA to look out for: jaw or tongue pain, jaw claudication, headache, scalp tenderness, and/or visual changes. Health literacy and rapid access to medical care may be important factors affecting how quickly ominous features of GCA may be acted on, and may partly explain why area-level socioeconomic deprivation is associated with ischaemic features at presentation of GCA (9).

15.3 Vascular stenosis

Although uncommon, progressive vascular stenosis may occur, especially in patients with the 'large-vessel' form of GCA who may not have cranial symptoms (10). Younger patients (<65 years) are at increased risk of this complication. Effective control of the inflammatory process prior to any vascular intervention is advisable. Control of the inflammation may improve the stenosis; fixed stenosis, presumably due to scarring, can be treated conservatively (exercise stimulates collateral formation) or with vascular intervention if necessary. During monitoring, all peripheral pulses should be examined and blood pressure should be measured in both arms.

15.4 Aortic complications

Aortic dilatation, aneurysm, dissection, and rupture are reported complications of GCA, with a 17-fold risk of thoracic aortic aneurysm and 2.4-fold risk of abdominal aortic aneurysm often quoted (11). However, UK general practitioner-coded data suggests only a twofold risk of aortic aneurysm overall; male sex, smoking, and hypertension were risk factors for developing an aneurysm in GCA, but diabetes appeared protective against aneurysm development, even though there was an association with susceptibility to GCA itself (12). Where cohorts of patients with GCA have been imaged systematically, one in five to ten patients may have an aortic aneurysm or dilatation (13), but not all of these patients go to surgery (14).

Dissection and rupture are commonest in the first year of GCA, suggesting that active inflammation is a risk factor. By contrast, aortic dilatation and aneurysm occur more gradually and may relate to destruction of the internal elastic lamina of the aorta, which normally provides the vascular wall with strength and elasticity (10). On current data there does not seem to be a positive association between risk of aneurysm/dilatation and intensity of the systemic inflammatory response (13).

15.5 Duration of glucocorticoid therapy

15.5.1 Typical durations

For PMR, glucocorticoids are titrated to symptoms whereas in GCA there is caution about reducing glucocorticoids over-quickly because of the potentially serious consequences of a relapse (15). Median duration of glucocorticoid therapy is usually around 2 years for isolated PMR (16) and for GCA (17). However, patients who develop PMR

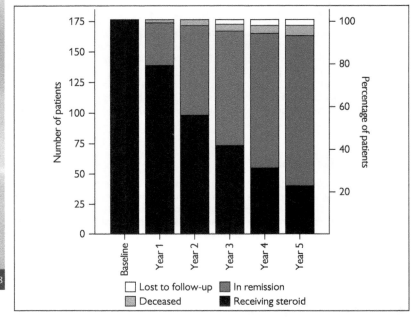

Figure 15.1 Duration of glucocorticoid therapy in PMR with 5-year follow-up.

Reproduced from Mackie SL, Hensor EM, Haugeberg G, Bhakta B, Pease CT: Can the prognosis of polymyalgia rheumatica be predicted at disease onset? Results from a 5-year prospective study. Rheumatology (Oxford, England) 2010, 49(4):716–722 with permission from Oxford University Press.

followed by GCA later tend to spend longer on glucocorticoids (16). In a Spanish cohort, two-thirds of GCA patients relapsed at least once, and one-third relapsed at least twice (7). The relapses usually happened during the first 2 years of treatment; those who relapsed had higher and more prolonged glucocorticoid requirements than those who did not relapse (Figure 15.1) (7). (See also Chapter 10.)

15.5.2 **Very prolonged treatment courses**

Some patients continue to take long-term glucocorticoids. Reasons are multifactorial; low-dose glucocorticoids can also ameliorate symptoms of other conditions such as osteoarthritis and rotator cuff lesions. In combination with iatrogenic adrenal suppression and/or steroid withdrawal symptoms, this may contribute to very prolonged treatment course.

15.5.3 **Recurrences**

Recurrences (the need to restart glucocorticoids after having been symptom free without treatment) are infrequent in PMR, but commoner in GCA (17). These recurrences may occur many years after the original episode.

15.6 **In polymyalgia rheumatica: onset of giant cell arteritis**

In population-based databases, 2–3% of patients diagnosed with PMR are diagnosed with GCA either on that day or later (18). In hospital-based cohorts the proportion is higher, up to 20%. Patients requiring higher initial doses of glucocorticoid may be more likely to develop GCA later (16). It might be speculated that some of these may have had subclinical GCA (perhaps LVV) from the start.

15.7 **In giant cell arteritis: onset of polymyalgia rheumatica**

In most reports, around half of GCA patients have associated polymyalgic symptoms. Some patients may not have prominent polymyalgic symptoms at presentation, but may develop these later during reduction of glucocorticoid dose, without a return of GCA symptoms. This prompts an increase in glucocorticoid dose, so that GCA patients with 'PMR relapses' usually are treated with glucocorticoids for longer than those without 'PMR relapses'.

15.8 **Tapering glucocorticoid therapy**

15.8.1 **Trade-offs**

It is a truism that patients who taper their glucocorticoid dose faster might be expected to stop glucocorticoids sooner, on average, but that they are likely to have a higher risk of disease relapse during the tapering. This trade-off is usually well understood by patients; patients frequently take an active role in contributing to decisions about how fast the dose should be tapered.

15.8.2 **Glucocorticoid withdrawal symptoms**

Over-fast glucocorticoid tapering can paradoxically lead to prolonged glucocorticoid therapy. This may in part relate to glucocorticoid withdrawal symptoms, which are particularly common in the first week after sudden reductions in dose, even at supraphysiological glucocorticoid doses. These withdrawal symptoms can include fatigue, myalgia, and headache, potentially mimicking PMR or GCA symptoms. This is one reason why tapering of the glucocorticoid dose tends to be more successful if carried out gradually.

15.8.3 **Adrenal suppression**

At glucocorticoid doses in the physiological range (<7.5 mg prednisolone), glucocorticoid tapering can be particularly difficult, as dose reduction may unmask iatrogenic adrenal suppression and cause adrenal insufficiency symptoms. In this scenario, very slow tapering may be helpful (19).

Because of the blunting of the cortisol component of the physiological stress response, it is generally advised that patients receiving long-term glucocorticoids at doses less than 15 mg may need supplementary glucocorticoid therapy during surgery or intercurrent illness. There have, however, been few studies investigating whether this is in fact beneficial.

15.9 **Female sex**

Two studies suggested that women with PMR may be at elevated risk of relapse and prolonged courses of therapy, compared to men with PMR (20, 21); however, not all studies have replicated this finding.

15.10 **Conclusion**

Although glucocorticoids provide very effective symptomatic relief in patients with PMR and GCA, long-term problems include complications of the disease (including cranial ischaemic complications, limb stenosis, and aortic complications) and the multiple potential complications of glucocorticoid treatment. It is important to provide holistic care for these patients in order to optimize prognosis.

References

1. Brack A, Martinez-Taboada V, Stanson A, et al. Disease pattern in cranial and large-vessel giant cell arteritis. Arthritis Rheum 1999; 42(2):311–17.

2. Prieto-Gonzalez S, Arguis P, Garcia-Martinez A, et al. Large vessel involvement in biopsy-proven giant cell arteritis: prospective study in 40 newly diagnosed patients using CT angiography. Ann Rheum Dis 2012; 71(7):1170–6.

3. Moosig F, Czech N, Mehl C, et al. Correlation between 18-fluorodeoxyglucose accumulation in large vessels and serological markers of inflammation in polymyalgia rheumatica: a quantitative PET study. Ann Rheum Dis 2004; 63(7):870–3.

4. Rao JK, Allen NB, Pincus T. Limitations of the 1990 American College of Rheumatology classification criteria in the diagnosis of vasculitis. Ann Intern Med 1998; 129(5):345–52.

5. Olivieri I, Pipitone N, D' Angelo S, et al. Late-onset rheumatoid arthritis and late-onset spondyloarthritis. Clin Exp Rheumatol 2009; 27(4 Suppl 55):S139–45.

6. Pease CT, Haugeberg G, Morgan AW, et al. Diagnosing late onset rheumatoid arthritis, polymyalgia rheumatica, and temporal arteritis in patients presenting with polymyalgic symptoms. A prospective longterm evaluation. J Rheumatol 2005; 32(6):1043–6.

7. Alba MA, Garcia-Martinez A, Prieto-Gonzalez S, et al. Relapses in patients with giant cell arteritis: prevalence, characteristics, and associated clinical findings in a longitudinally followed cohort of 106 patients. Medicine 2014; 93(5):194–201.

8. Nesher G, Berkun Y, Mates M, et al. Low-dose aspirin and prevention of cranial ischemic complications in giant cell arteritis. Arthritis Rheum 2004; 50(4):1332–7.

9. Mackie SL, Dasgupta B, Hordon L, et al. Ischaemic manifestations in giant cell arteritis are associated with area level socio-economic deprivation, but not cardiovascular risk factors. Rheumatology (Oxford) 2011; 50(11):2014–22.

10. Nuenninghoff DM, Hunder GG, Christianson TJ, et al. Incidence and predictors of large-artery complication (aortic aneurysm, aortic dissection, and/or large-artery stenosis) in patients with giant cell arteritis: a population-based study over 50 years. Arthritis Rheum 2003; 48(12):3522–31.

11. Evans JM, O'Fallon WM, Hunder GG. Increased incidence of aortic aneurysm and dissection in giant cell (temporal) arteritis. A population-based study. Ann Intern Med 1995; 122(7):502–7.

12. Robson JC, Kiran A, Maskell J, et al. The relative risk of aortic aneurysm in patients with giant cell arteritis compared with the general population of the UK. Ann Rheum Dis 2015; 74(1):129–35.

13. Mackie SL, Hensor EM, Morgan AW, et al. Should I send my patient with previous giant cell arteritis for imaging of the thoracic aorta? A systematic literature review and meta-analysis. Ann Rheum Dis 2014; 73(1):143–8.

14. Garcia-Martinez A, Arguis P, Prieto-Gonzalez S, et al. Prospective long term follow-up of a cohort of patients with giant cell arteritis screened for aortic structural damage (aneurysm or dilatation). Ann Rheum Dis 2014; 73(10):1826–32.

15. Mukhtyar C, Guillevin L, Cid MC, et al. EULAR recommendations for the management of large vessel vasculitis. Ann Rheum Dis 2009; 68(3):318–23.

16. Mackie SL, Hensor EM, Haugeberg G, *et al.* Can the prognosis of polymyalgia rheumatica be predicted at disease onset? Results from a 5-year prospective study. *Rheumatology (Oxford)* 2010; 49(4):716–22.

17. Proven A, Gabriel SE, Orces C, *et al.* Glucocorticoid therapy in giant cell arteritis: duration and adverse outcomes. *Arthritis Rheum* 2003; 49(5):703–8.

18. Smeeth L, Cook C, Hall AJ. Incidence of diagnosed polymyalgia rheumatica and temporal arteritis in the United Kingdom, 1990–2001. *Ann Rheum Dis* 2006; 65(8):1093–8.

19. Patt H, Bandgar T, Lila A, *et al.* Management issues with exogenous steroid therapy. *Indian J Endocrinol Metab* 2013; 17(Suppl 3):S612–17.

20. Cimmino MA, Parodi M, Caporali R, *et al.* Is the course of steroid-treated polymyalgia rheumatica more severe in women? *Ann N Y Acad Sci* 2006; 1069:315–21.

21. Barraclough K, Liddell WG, du Toit J, *et al.* Polymyalgia rheumatica in primary care: a cohort study of the diagnostic criteria and outcome. *Fam Pract* 2008; 25(5):328–33.

Chapter 16

Primary care

Toby Helliwell, Samantha L. Hider, and Christian D. Mallen

Key points

- Polymyalgia rheumatica (PMR) is the commonest inflammatory rheumatological disorder of older people, causing significant pain and stiffness of the shoulders and hips.
- Giant cell arteritis (GCA) is the commonest form of large-vessel vasculitis and needs urgent assessment to prevent serious complications, including permanent visual loss.
- Initial symptoms of both may be non-specific; therefore diagnosis in primary care remains challenging and requires a systematic approach to exclude other potential causes of pathology.
- Treatment with glucocorticoids is successful for most patients but requires careful monitoring of potential adverse events.
- Long-term management of both conditions can occur in primary care.

133

16.1 Introduction

PMR and GCA are both inflammatory disorders of older people that present significant diagnostic and management challenges to primary clinicians. This chapter presents the primary care epidemiology and clinical presentation of PMR and GCA, highlighting the best current evidence-based practice for the diagnosis, treatment, and long-term monitoring of these disabling and often suboptimally managed conditions.

16.2 Epidemiology in primary care

One of the most widely used estimates of the incidence of both PMR and GCA comes from a large primary care-based study (1). Using validated electronic consultation data from the UK General Practice Research Database, Smeeth et al. (1) report the overall age-adjusted incidence rate of PMR at 8.4/10,000 person years (with a female-to-male ratio of 2.0) in primary care consultations, whilst the overall age-adjusted incidence rate of GCA was reported as 2.2/10,000 person years (with a female-to-male ratio of 2.6).

With the increase in life expectancy, the number of patients suffering from PMR and GCA being encountered in primary care is set to rise.

16.3 **Polymyalgia rheumatica**

In the United Kingdom, the majority of PMR patients are managed exclusively in primary care (2, 3) with around 15% of patients being referred to secondary care for diagnosis (3). The average full-time GP will see four new cases of PMR per year with a practice with 10,000 patients recording 20 consultations per year for PMR (4) making this an important condition for primary care health professionals to be aware of.

16.3.1 **Making the diagnosis**

Making the diagnosis of PMR and GCA can be challenging, even for specialists (5). Patients presenting with classical symptoms who have a good response to low-dose glucocorticoids can be safely managed in the community; however, atypical presentations are not unusual and as such, vigilance is needed in making the diagnosis. Symptoms, such as joint pain, stiffness, and fatigue are common in primary care and as such, a systematic approach to diagnosis is essential to eliminate other disorders with overlapping symptoms.

UK PMR management guidelines (6, 7) identify a number of serious disorders that can mimic PMR and in some cases, symptoms may initially respond to low-dose glucocorticoids. Accurate diagnosis is therefore essential, both to ensure that other diagnoses are not missed and to ensure that potential adverse events resulting from inappropriate glucocorticoid treatment are avoided. In cases of diagnostic uncertainty, early referral for specialist review is essential. Some examples of indications for early referral for PMR are summarized in Box 16.1. Ongoing management can usually continue in primary care once diagnosis has been confirmed, although specialist input should be considered if the steroid response is poor or there are recurrent symptom relapses (6).

16.3.2 **Treatment dilemmas**

Whilst the majority of patients with PMR exhibit a dramatic response to low-dose treatment with glucocorticoids, up to 20% of patients remain symptomatic. This group should be referred to specialist services to re-examine the diagnosis of PMR and to consider alternative treatment options. Other indications for referral to secondary care are provided in Box 16.2.

16.4 **Giant cell arteritis**

Diagnosing GCA can be difficult. The average GP will only see one new case every 1–2 years and the low sensitivity of presenting features makes recognition, especially of non-typical presentations, challenging (7, 8).

Box 16.1 Indications for early specialist review

- Age less than 60 years
- Chronic onset
- Lack of shoulder involvement
- Lack of inflammatory stiffness
- Red flag features (prominent systemic features, weight loss, abnormal neurology)
- Features of peripheral inflammatory arthritis or muscle disease, other autoimmune/ systemic diseases
- Very high or normal inflammatory markers.

> Box 16.2 Common treatment dilemmas needing specialist referral
>
> • Contraindications to glucocorticoid therapy
> • Poor/incomplete response to glucocorticoids
> • Inability to reduce glucocorticoid therapy
> • Recurrent relapses
> • Prolonged treatment duration (>2 years)
> • Occurrence of glucocorticoid-related adverse events.

Only half of all patients with GCA present with the classical temporal headache and only around a third have scalp tenderness or jaw symptoms (9). Unfortunately, headache as a presenting feature is over-relied upon and patients with GCA without headache are at high risk of developing irreversible visual loss owing to delayed diagnosis (10, 11).

All patients with suspected GCA should be referred to specialist services, ideally using a fast-track referral pathway enabling rapid assessment (11). Different areas have different pathways involving different specialties (e.g. rheumatology, ophthalmology, geriatrics, and vascular surgery) and as such, it is prudent to familiarize yourself with the locally available care pathways and to lobby for rapid access clinics that have direct access to specialists experienced in performing investigations including temporal artery ultrasound and biopsy if not already provided.

Patients with suspected GCA should be treated *immediately* (prior to being seen in a specialist setting) with high-dose glucocorticoids to avoid potentially serious complications. In the absence of ischaemic symptoms (jaw claudication or visual symptoms), current guidance is to initiate treatment with 40–60 mg prednisolone per day. The risk of visual complications is higher in patients with jaw claudication and as such, this group should be prescribed a higher dose (usually 60 mg prednisolone/day) (7). For patients already experiencing visual symptoms (e.g. amaurosis fugax), immediate expert help should be searched for because intravenous methylprednisolone may be used (7, 8).

16.5 **Monitoring and management of comorbidities**

A key role for primary care clinicians is regular monitoring of patients including the assessment of the accuracy of the original diagnosis, checking for relapses (which are common), and investigating/treating glucocorticoid-related complications. In particular, patients with PMR should be educated about and assessed regularly for GCA symptoms.

Adverse events potentially related to glucocorticoid treatment are common in patients with PMR and GCA (12) and are a major concern to patients (13). Most relevant adverse effects include weight gain, bruising, infections, glaucoma, myopathy, osteoporosis, diabetes, hypertension, depression, and dyspepsia. Patients should be provided with a steroid information card and be fully informed about potential side effects.

A key role for primary care is to prevent and manage multimorbidity in patients with PMR and GCA. Gastroprotection with a proton pump inhibitor should be considered, especially in older patients or those with a history of gastrointestinal comorbidity. Patients with GCA should be started on prophylaxis with calcium, vitamin D, and bisphosphonates in view of the potentially high risk of osteoporosis. Patients with PMR

- Polymyalgia Rheumatica and Giant Cell Arteritis UK (PMRGCAuk; http://www.pmrgcauk.com/)—provides information on PMR and GCA, peer support from patients, and a telephone helpline
- Arthritis Research UK (http://www.arthritisresearchuk.org/arthritis-information/conditions/polymyalgia-rheumatica.aspx and http://www.arthritisresearchuk.org/arthritis-information/conditions/giant-cell-arteritis.aspx)—provides written information on the diagnosis and treatment of PMR and GCA
- Patient (http://www.patient.info/health/polymyalgia-rheumatica and http://www.patient.info/doctor/giant-cell-arteritis-temporal-arteritis-pro)—useful information on the diagnosis and treatment (and treatment side effects) of PMR and GCA.

should be started on calcium and vitamin D, and bisphosphonates added if the fracture risk is high (e.g. FRAX® assessment). For high-risk patients, a baseline dual-energy X-ray absorptiometry scan should be arranged if indicated (6, 14).

Blood pressure and serum glucose should be monitored, especially in patients with pre-existing hypertension and diabetes. Data suggest that patients with PMR and GCA have an increased risk for cardiovascular disease (15, 16) and thus screening for and aggressive management of vascular risk factors is warranted. Advice on smoking cessation, exercise, and remaining physically active is also important.

16.6 **Patient education and counselling**

Primary care has a critical role in patient education and counselling for patients with PMR and GCA. The provision of high-quality written information is an essential part of the patient journey. Evidence suggests that not only do patients want access to high-quality educational resources, but also that patient information can help to improve medical outcomes and reduce anxiety and concerns. Several quality resources exist for patients with PMR and GCA (see Box 16.3).

References

1. Smeeth L, Cook C, Hall AJ. Incidence of diagnosed polymyalgia rheumatica and temporal arteritis in the United Kingdom, 1990–2001. *Ann Rheum Dis* 2006; 65(8):1093–8.

2. Helliwell T, Hider SL, Mallen CD. Polymyalgia rheumatica: diagnosis, prescribing, and monitoring in general practice. *Br J Gen Pract* 2013; 63(610):e361–6.

3. Barraclough K, Liddell WG, du Toit J, et al. Polymyalgia rheumatica in primary care: a cohort study of the diagnostic criteria and outcome. *Fam Pract* 2008; 25(5):328–33.

4. Arthritis Research UK National Primary Care Centre. Consultations for selected diagnoses and regional problems. In *Musculoskeletal Matters Bulletin No. 2*. [Online] http://www.keele.ac.uk/media/keeleuniversity/ri/primarycare/bulletins/MusculoskeletalMatters2.pdf

5. Dasgupta B, Cimmino MA, Maradit-Kremers H, et al. 2012 provisional classification criteria for polymyalgia rheumatica: a European League Against Rheumatism/American College of Rheumatology collaborative initiative. *Ann Rheum Dis* 2012; 71(4):484–92.

6. Dasgupta B, Borg FA, Hassan N, et al. BSR and BHPR guidelines for the management of polymyalgia rheumatica. *Rheumatology (Oxford)* 2010; 49:186–90.

7. Dasgupta B, Borg FA, Hassan N, *et al*. BSR and BHPR guidelines for the management of giant cell arteritis. *Rheumatology (Oxford)* 2010; 49(8):1594–7.

8. Barraclough K, Mallen CD, Helliwell T, *et al*. Diagnosis and management of giant cell arteritis. *Br J Gen Pract* 2012; 62(599):329–30.

9. Smetana GW, Shmerling RH. Does this patient have temporal arteritis? *JAMA* 2002; 287(1): 92–101.

10. Ezeonyeji AN, Borg FA, Dasgupta B. Delays in recognition and management of giant cell arteritis: results from a retrospective audit. *Clin Rheumatol* 2011; 30(2):259–62.

11. Patil P, Williams M, Maw WW, *et al*. Fast track pathway reduces sight loss in giant cell arteritis: results of a longitudinal observational cohort study. *Clin Exp Rheumatol* 2015; 33(2 Suppl 89):S103–6.

12. Mazzantini M, Torre C, Miccoli M, *et al*. Adverse events during longterm low-dose glucocorticoid treatment of polymyalgia rheumatica: a retrospective study. *J Rheumatol* 2012; 39(3):552–7.

13. Mackie SL, Arat S, da Silva J, *et al*. Polymyalgia Rheumatica (PMR) Special Interest Group at OMERACT 11: outcomes of importance for patients with PMR. *J Rheumatol* 2014; 41(4):819–23.

14. Mackie SL, Mallen CD. Polymyalgia rheumatica. *BMJ* 2013; 347:f6937.

15. Hancock AT, Mallen CD, Belcher J, *et al*. Association between polymyalgia rheumatica and vascular disease: a systematic review. *Arthritis Care Res (Hoboken)* 2012; 64(9):1301–5.

16. Hancock AT, Mallen CD, Muller S, *et al*. Risk of vascular events in patients with polymyalgia rheumatica. *CMAJ* 2014; 186(13):E495–501.

Chapter 17

Socioeconomic implications

Matthew J. Koster, Eric L. Matteson, and Cynthia S. Crowson

Key points

- Utilization and medical cost is highest among polymyalgia rheumatica (PMR) patients in the first year following diagnosis.
- Diagnosis of PMR/giant cell arteritis (GCA) and management of treatment-related side effects account for the majority of associated healthcare expenditures.
- Limited epidemiological information is available on the socioeconomic impact of PMR/GCA and further research is necessary.

17.1 Introduction

Whereas the socioeconomic impacts of osteoarthritis, rheumatoid arthritis, and systemic lupus erythematosus have been well described (1–5), research focused on the socioeconomic implications of other rheumatic diseases is scarce. Despite the well-recognized severity, duration, and complications of the systemic vasculitides, few studies have directly evaluated the healthcare utilization, cost, and economic burden of these diseases. Relative rarity, difficulty in obtaining valid population-based incidence and prevalence estimates, and insufficient databases available to address healthcare cost across all payer systems have contributed to incomplete evaluation of this area. The current limited knowledge regarding the socioeconomic implications of PMR and GCA will be reviewed here.

There are three major domains of direct medical costs related to GCA and PMR: (1) establishing a diagnosis, (2) treatment of active disease, and (3) management of late-stage disease and treatment-related complications.

17.2 Establishing a diagnosis

Difficulty in establishing the diagnosis of PMR can lead to substantial utilization of health-care resources and increased cost. A retrospective chart review of 123 PMR patients referred to a tertiary Canadian rheumatology clinic demonstrated that only 24% of patients were correctly identified as PMR by family physicians at time of referral (6). The mean cost of investigations to establish a diagnosis prior to referral was 3.8 times higher than the consensus estimate cost of diagnosing uncomplicated PMR advocated by local rheumatologists. This study provides evidence that educational programmes on the presentation, evaluation, and timely referral of patients with rheumatic diseases,

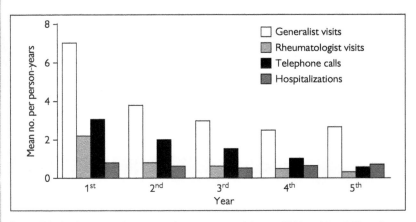

Figure 17.1 Health services utilization over the entire course of disease of 364 residents of Olmsted County, MN, USA (≥ 50 years of age) who first fulfilled the diagnostic criteria for polymyalgia rheumatica between 1970 and 2000.

Reproduced from Kremers HM, Reinalda MS, Crowson CS, Zinsmeister AR, Hunder GG, Gabriel SE., Use of physician services in a population-based cohort of patients with polymyalgia rheumatica over the course of their disease, 2005, with permission from Wiley.

including PMR, are needed to assist in effective diagnosis and cost containment. It also makes the economic case for early referral to the rheumatologist for confirmation of the diagnosis in most cases of PMR. After a diagnosis has been established, patients with PMR demonstrate considerable utilization of medical resources. A population-based cohort of 364 incident cases of PMR followed for a mean duration of 4.1 years showed that this group utilized 5108 physician office visits and 2015 telephone calls (7). The highest proportion of care occurred in the year immediately following diagnosis with 70% of all physician visits and 61% of all rheumatologist visits occurring within the first year of disease. The mean number of generalist visits observed per person-year of follow-up was 7.0 during the first year, 3.8 during the second year, and 3 or fewer visits thereafter (Figure 17.1). Rheumatologist visits were 2.2, 0.8, and 0.6 or fewer visits per person-year over the same intervals. Not unexpectedly, patients with PMR who developed GCA, had at least one relapse, or experienced corticosteroid complications required more rheumatologist visits than those without these outcomes.

17.3 **Treatment of active disease**

Direct medical costs of treating PMR have only been addressed in one population-based study observing 193 patients with PMR compared to 695 age- and sex-matched control subjects without PMR (8). The total yearly cost (inflation-adjusted to 2002 US dollars) of care for PMR was highest during the first year following diagnosis with a median cost of $2814 (interquartile range $1423–6820) and then was constant at approximately $1500/year. In contrast, cost for medical care among non-PMR subjects was relatively stable at $1000/year throughout the study duration (Figure 17.2). Over 5 years following diagnosis, the incremental cost of PMR was $2233 at the 10th percentile and $27,712 at the 90th percentile of cost. Within this population, subjects with PMR were nearly twice as likely to have other co-morbidities including myocardial infarction, peripheral vascular disease, and cerebrovascular disease than comparator

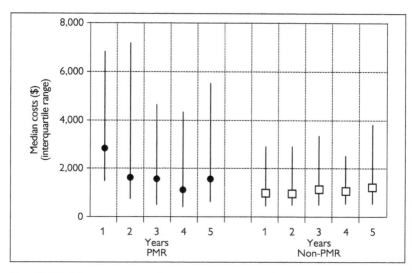

Figure 17.2 Total direct medical costs of care by years of follow-up (inflation-adjusted to 2002 US dollars). Subjects censored in a particular year were not included in the calculation of median costs in subsequent years. PMR, polymyalgia rheumatica.

Reproduced from Kremers HM, Reinalda MS, Crowson CS, Zinsmeister AR, Hunder GG, Gabriel SE., Direct medical costs of polymyalgia rheumatica, 2005, with permission from Wiley.

subjects; adjustment for such co-morbidities attenuated the incremental cost difference between PMR subjects and controls. Whether these specific vascular comorbidities can be directly attributable to PMR itself, treatment with corticosteroids, or another aetiology remains under debate (9–11).

The majority of evaluation and management of patients with GCA occurs in the outpatient setting. In spite of this, information regarding outpatient utilization and cost is not currently available for GCA. Cotch and colleagues (12) evaluated hospitalizations in 1986–1990 among patients with five selected vasculitis conditions in New York State, United States. GCA comprised 59% of the 5942 vasculitis patients identified and accounted for 4518 hospitalizations over the 5-year study period. The total calculated cost for hospitalizations among patients with GCA in New York State was $28.4 million. Extrapolating to the entire United States, the cost of hospitalizations among patients with GCA was estimated to be $355.4 million in 1986–1990.

17.4 **Management of late-stage disease and treatment-related complications**

In addition to cost related to diagnosis and initial treatment for PMR and GCA, a substantial economic burden stems from associated co-morbidities and treatment-related side effects. A recent report predicted cost of visual impairment secondary to GCA, which occurs in up to 20% of patients, and the financial effect of corticosteroid-induced fracture. If current incidences and treatment strategies remain unchanged, over the next 35 years a projected 140,000 patients with GCA in the United States will present with acute visual symptoms requiring hospital admission and treatment, accounting for

$1.13 billion in inpatient management and $70.63 billion in cumulative cost for visually impaired patients (13). Additional co-morbidities of large-vessel vasculitis and aortic complications have yet to be investigated.

Up to 59% of patients with PMR (14) and 90% of patients with GCA (15) experience at least one corticosteroid-associated complication, the most frequent being corticosteroid-induced osteoporotic bone fracture. By 2050, 360,000 patients with GCA in the United States are projected to develop a corticosteroid-induced fracture with an estimated cost of management over $6.5 billion (13). Current or projected costs of other known corticosteroid-associated complications including hypertension, cataracts, diabetes mellitus, infection, and avascular necrosis have not been calculated.

17.5 **Summary**

In summary, patients with PMR and GCA exhibit a high utilization of healthcare services and cost, most notably in the year following diagnosis. These conditions require long-term treatment with corticosteroids, which are associated with significant morbidity. While the life expectancy of patients with PMR and GCA is generally not different from that of people without GCA or PMR, complications of the disease, especially early visual loss, and complications of sometimes catastrophic vascular complications such as aortic aneurysms and arterial stenosis, pose a major burden on the individual patient, the healthcare system, and society. The full impact of these diseases on societal cost is unknown and requires further study. Emphasis on appropriate diagnostic evaluations, timely referrals, and mitigation of disease-related and treatment-related complications provide opportunities to decrease the observed economic burden. The implications of changes in assessment of disease activity (e.g. ultrasound and advanced imaging such as magnetic resonance imaging, computed tomography, and positron emission tomography for disease diagnosis and activity assessment) or treatment (e.g. corticosteroid-sparing strategies) of PMR and GCA are not yet known.

References

1. Carls G, Li T, Panopalis P, et al. Direct and indirect costs to employers of patients with systemic lupus erythematosus with and without nephritis. J Occup Environ Med 2009; 51(1):66–79.

2. Lau CS, Mak A. The socioeconomic burden of SLE. Nat Rev Rheumatol 2009; 5(7):400–4.

3. Panopalis P, Clarke AE, Yelin E. The economic burden of systemic lupus erythematosus. Best Pract Res Clin Rheumatol 2012; 26(5):695–704.

4. Furneri G, Mantovani LG, Belisari A, et al. Systematic literature review on economic implications and pharmacoeconomic issues of rheumatoid arthritis. Clin Exp Rheumatol 2012; 30(4 Suppl 73):S72–84.

5. Gabriel SE, Crowson CS, Campion ME, et al. Direct medical costs unique to people with arthritis. J Rheumatol 1997; 24(4):719–25.

6. Bahlas S, Ramos-Remus C, Davis P. Utilisation and costs of investigations, and accuracy of diagnosis of polymyalgia rheumatica by family physicians. Clin Rheumatol 2000; 19(4):278–80.

7. Kremers HM, Reinalda MS, Crowson CS, et al. Use of physician services in a population-based cohort of patients with polymyalgia rheumatica over the course of their disease. Arthritis Rheum 2005; 53(3):395–403.

8. Kremers HM, Reinalda MS, Crowson CS, et al. Direct medical costs of polymyalgia rheumatica. Arthritis Rheum 2005; 53(4):578–84.

9. Mazzantini M, Torre C, Miccoli M, *et al.* Adverse events during longterm low-dose gluco-corticoid treatment of polymyalgia rheumatica: a retrospective study. *J Rheumatol* 2012; 39(3):552–7.

10. Maradit Kremers H, Reinalda MS, Crowson CS, *et al.* Glucocorticoids and cardiovascular and cerebrovascular events in polymyalgia rheumatica. *Arthritis Rheum* 2007; 57(2):279–86.

11. Bartoloni E, Alunno A, Santoboni G, *et al.* Beneficial cardiovascular effects of low-dose gluco-corticoid therapy in inflammatory rheumatic diseases. *J Rheumatol* 2012; 39(8):1758–60.

12. Cotch MFH, Gary S. The prevalence, epidemiology and cost of hospitalizations for vasculitis in New York State 1986 to 1990. *Arthritis Rheum* 1995; 38(9):S225.

13. De Smit E, Palmer AJ, Hewitt AW. Projected worldwide disease burden from giant cell arte-ritis by 2050. *J Rheumatol* 2015; 42:119–25.

14. Kremers HM, Reinalda MS, Crowson CS, *et al.* Relapse in a population based cohort of patients with polymyalgia rheumatica. *J Rheumatol* 2005; 32(1):65–73.

15. Dunstan E, Lester SL, Rischmueller M, *et al.* Epidemiology of biopsy-proven giant cell arteritis in South Australia. *Intern Med J* 2014; 44(1):32–9.

Chapter 18

Patient education

Kate Gilbert

Key points

- Polymyalgia rheumatica (PMR) is little known and poorly understood in lay circles. Newly diagnosed patients may feel a strong need to connect with someone with personal experience of the condition. Such support is readily provided by patient organizations such as PMRGCAuk, by means of support groups, online forums, helplines, and social media.

- At diagnosis and as treatment proceeds, clinicians should ensure that patients know how to contact a patient organization. During tapering of steroids, patient needs shift from information to support with the symptomatic effects of steroid reduction.

- Every PMR patient should have information about the cardinal signs and symptoms of giant cell arteritis.

18.1 Learning points of this chapter

This chapter outlines the importance of patient education for the successful management of PMR and giant cell arteritis (GCA). Sources of information and support are presented, with contact details and a review of the type of support available.

18.2 Introduction

Most people who develop PMR or GCA have, on diagnosis, never heard of either condition. Many will have struggled for months with painful and disabling symptoms, fearing the worst. So when they get a diagnosis of something they have never heard of, they may well feel some sense of relief that they apparently do not have a life-threatening illness, but they will also feel confusion and frustration. They hear the word 'steroids' and immediately fantasize about the side effects of the medication. Some will initially reject the idea of medication altogether, and it can be difficult for doctors to persuade them that they need to take prednisolone not only to control their symptoms, but to protect their eyesight. Actually, in a small-scale survey of PMR patients carried out by PMRGCAuk, it was found that over 50% of newly diagnosed patients were not informed at all by their general practitioner (GP) about the connection between PMR and GCA, and the concomitant threat to eyesight. Similarly, almost 60% of patients are not informed by their doctors, either GPs or rheumatologists, of the effect of glucocorticosteroids on raising blood sugars. Patient education is a key issue in the management of PMR and GCA, and the role of patient-led voluntary organizations is paramount in presenting this information in a way which people can absorb and understand when they are both in the acute stages of their illness and the long 'tail' of reducing their level of corticosteroids.

However, patient education begins in the surgery at diagnosis with the clinician, and needs follow-up as the patient proceeds through the course of their illness. The patient should be fully informed about PMR/GCA and the treatment required, the normal duration of treatment, and the patient involvement in the whole process. This will enhance the path of shared decision-making between the patient and doctor.

Not only does the patient require corticosteroid therapy and bone protection, they will need to understand the difference between inflammatory PMR muscle pain and mechanical pain. The patient will learn to distinguish between the two and know when they are 'flaring' and when they are not.

The patient may have other co-morbidities which will need to be taken into consideration at diagnosis (e.g. osteoporosis, diabetes, or hypertension). Therefore a detailed history is required along with an individualized written management plan agreed by the patient at the beginning of treatment. The management plan will be discussed and amended when required, depending on the needs of the patient.

Physical exercise is also very important and the involvement of a physiotherapist may be required to maintain range of movement and general fitness levels. Quality of rest may also improve well-being and recovery, and a physiotherapist may be able to advise on this (e.g. by giving information on a healthy sleeping position). Eating well and maintaining a healthy lifestyle is extremely important as steroid therapy has long-term side effects. Educating the patient and discussing diet, exercise, prevention of osteoporosis, and maintaining a healthy weight will be necessary along with routine eye tests at the local optician and GP blood pressure monitoring during treatment. This will highlight any abnormalities early.

18.3 Getting and giving support

It is widely acknowledged that patient-led support initiatives can help to improve patient self-efficacy in managing long-term conditions (1). In England, PMRGCAuk and its local support groups, and in Scotland, PMR and GCA Scotland, are providing helpline services and sending out information packs to people who are newly diagnosed and those some way into treatment.

18.4 Helplines

An advice line for patients is a vital service whether it is via the GP practice or the rheumatology clinic. The patient will be able to discuss any concerns about their treatment and get prompt appropriate advice from a knowledgeable medical resource. This will help to ensure that steroid therapy is given at the right dose and not increased/decreased for the wrong reason. In turn, it will reassure patients that they have professional support when they are in need.

PMRGCAuk and the other organizations listed below reinforce the information and support the patient through their journey, both at the end of a telephone and face-to-face at a support group, adding the additional dimension of personal experience.

Helpline and group volunteers all either have, or have had, PMR or GCA and thus have personal experience of the issues that sufferers are dealing with on a daily basis.

The first thing that brought people together to form the group that would become PMRGCAuk, was the need for a national helpline (2). The founders of the charity wanted there to be help at the end of the telephone for anybody, whether they needed information, reassurance, or just a listening ear.

PMRGCAuk launched its helpline in January 2011. That month, there were 20 calls. At the time of writing (2015) there are around 100 per month. People can call for all sorts of reasons, but they tend to fall into three main types. The first type is from people who have just been diagnosed, who want more information. Often their GPs have printed out information in the surgery and sent them home to read through it, and they have found the name of the charity. We can give these callers information (but not so much that they are overloaded, because they need time to absorb it) and some reassurance that they will start feeling better soon. We check that patients are aware of the danger of damage to their sight if PMR flares up into GCA, and how to recognize the symptoms. We try to send out an information pack as soon as possible. The information pack contains the relevant booklet (3, 4), our newsletter, information about membership and services provided by PMRGCAuk, and a list of support groups. For more complex situations, we may also include the relevant British Society for Rheumatology guidelines.

The second type of call is from people who are quite a long way into their PMR or GCA journey and are having trouble tapering the dose of steroids. GPs and information leaflets tend to give the impression that lowering the dose and coming off prednisolone is a fairly smooth and trouble-free process. Maybe it is for some, but too many find it extremely challenging, and they wonder if they are the only people who are suffering so. They even start to blame themselves for not being able to come off. They need to know that their experience is not weird: it is typical.

Another group of callers are those, often quite elderly, people who have been stricken with PMR or GCA on top of other long-term conditions. They may already be taking complicated combinations of drugs and are worried about the way in which both their 'new' illness, and the prednisolone, might affect their pre-existing conditions. For volunteers it can be a challenge because, however much we try to read and understand some of the science behind PMR and GCA diagnosis and treatment, none of us is medically qualified, and we have to explain that we cannot give clinical advice. However, most people find it really helpful just to share their concerns with somebody who is a good listener and understands a bit about what they have been going through. Almost everyone says, at the end of a call, that it was great to talk with somebody who has, or has had, this peculiar illness.

Occasionally we have had calls from people who we have had to tell to call a taxi and get themselves to hospital in case they have GCA. Fortunately this doesn't happen terribly often because, by and large, people come to the helpline after they have been diagnosed and generally after they have started treatment.

The volunteers on the helpline do not have medical qualifications, but we have a set of guidelines and procedures that they are required to follow. There is also recourse to a Medical Advisory Panel composed of specialist rheumatologists, researchers, a physiotherapist, an ophthalmologist, and a pharmacist. PMRGCAuk is a member of The Helplines Association and follow their good practice guidelines, so that callers will have the reassurance of quality of the service. Callers may be referred to the Arthritis Care helpline, which is manned by highly trained professional staff with immediate access to a vast bank of information. Callers who are beyond the competence of the

PMR and GCA volunteers on the PMRGCAuk helpline, for example, because of other pre-existing serious and chronic conditions, are thus referred to Arthritis Care for further information and support.

18.5 Support groups

The first support group in England was set up by a patient in East Anglia in 2004. This was closely followed by a group in Southend. Around about the same time, a group became established in Dundee, which later became PMR and GCA Scotland. In 2008, Professor Dasgupta brought these groups together, along with a group of patients who had met on the Internet forum at Patient.info, to form a working party to establish the national charity.

Most of the groups meet regularly, although not frequently. All support groups are patient led and owe their existence to the efforts and energies of determined PMR and GCA sufferers who want to help other people in a similar position to themselves.

Groups offer a range of activities, from guest speakers such as the local consultant rheumatologist, to movement sessions with physiotherapists, and contributions from alternative therapists. Clinicians find that the time they spend attending a group meeting to speak is a great way to give out information, and learn from patients. A group situation can often increase and improve overall levels of communication. It is good for consultants to see their patients outside the clinical setting, to see them as whole people with families and a place in the community. An essential feature, though, is the support, solidarity, understanding, and acceptance that people with PMR and GCA can share with each other. Support groups undoubtedly give good value. For example, PMRGCAuk's 2012 survey found that 91% of respondents in support groups agreed that it was helpful to meet other people in the same position in person, whereas 86% found the contributions of speakers valuable, helping them to manage their condition (5). It was interesting to learn that 83% said that leaders of the group also provided support through phone contact. This is in addition to the services provided by the PMRGCAuk helpline.

Successful as the network of groups is, there are still huge gaps around the United Kingdom. As with the helpline, PMRGCAuk is always on the lookout for people who can help set up and run groups. Key clinical colleagues, such as rheumatology nurses, can give invaluable initial support in this process, discussing the possibility of a group with patients, and liaising with the charity and a local volunteer to get the initial meeting off the ground. Most groups become self-supporting after one or two meetings.

No doubt PMRGCAuk is no different from other health charities in finding that its network of support groups is valuable for sufferers of chronic health conditions; but there are some features that make our groups extraordinary. The first is that the average age of members of PMRGCAuk is about 76 years. It is quite something for a person who has PMR or GCA themselves, perhaps well into their 60s, to set up and manage a group for other people, and for elderly people to make huge efforts, as they do, to travel many miles in some cases to their regular group meeting. One thing that might be an incentive is that group members get to meet people at different stages of their illness. Those newly diagnosed can learn what may be facing them in the future (good and bad) and those further on in their 'journey' can see how far they have come. In the earlier-mentioned survey, seven out of ten group members said that being part of

Organization	Website	Helpline	Web forum	Newsletter
PMRGCAuk	http://www.pmrgcauk.com	0300 111 5090	http://healthunlocked.com/pmrgcauk	3/year
PMR and GCA Scotland	http://www.pmrandgca.org.uk	0300 777 5090	As above	As above
PMR-GCA UK North East Support	http://www.pmr-gca-northeast.org.uk		http://pmrandgca.forumup.co.uk	
Arthritis Research UK	http://www.arthritisresearchuk.org			
Arthritis Care	http://www.arthritiscare.org.uk	0808 800 4050	http://www.arthritiscareforum.org.uk/	4/year
Vasculitis UK	http://www.vasculitis.org.uk	0300 365 0075	http://www.healthunlocked.com/vasculitis-uk	2/year
Patient UK	http://www.patient.info		http://www.patient.info/forums	

Table 18.1 Summary table of relevant voluntary organizations

the group made them feel more optimistic about their prospects for recovery. This just shows how important it is to reduce the sense of isolation.

18.6 **Web forums**

In 2011, PMRGCAuk trustees agreed to an experimental trial period with an online organization, HealthUnlocked, who provide a 'platform' for health-related organizations to create virtual communities of people with chronic conditions. There is no doubt that older PMR and GCA sufferers are unlikely to be regular users of the Internet, or see it as a source of information and support. This is changing and we can anticipate that within the next 10 years, most older people will be active online. The community now has over 1000 members. People can post questions about any aspect of their experience with PMR and/or GCA, and other members are free to give advice, information, or encouragement. PMRGCAuk volunteers have a role in moderating what happens on the forum. Other organizations also run relevant forums, as shown in Table 18.1.

Being a member of the web forum is great for people who have complex health conditions running alongside their PMR or GCA. For example, people with heart conditions that predate their PMR or GCA, who have concerns about the cocktail of medications they are taking; and people who are unlucky enough to get shingles because they are on methotrexate, which has suppressed their immune system. They can almost always get a response to their questions from somebody who has either been in the same position or knows something about it. Many of the members say that they get more information from the forum than from anywhere else.

This does raise the issue of the role of self-appointed 'experts' on a patient-led information and education service, especially given the fact that research reports are now universally available on sites such as Medscape. Some 'activist' sufferers become so knowledgeable about the illnesses that they are more 'expert' on PMR or GCA, or on the risks and benefits of various forms of treatment, that it is not an exaggeration to say that, at least on a superficial level, they know more than most GPs.

18.7 **Patient education action checklist**

- Print off information for the patient from http://www.patient.info. Add PMRGCAuk helpline number 0300 111 5090 at the bottom.
- If the patient has suspected GCA, print out a copy of the information leaflet on temporal artery biopsy from http://www.pmrgca.co.uk/downloads/2/10
- Encourage the patient to ask PMRGCAuk for an info pack. If the patient cannot do this, please ask the surgery to email info@pmrgcauk.com with the patient's name and address and ask for the info pack to be posted out. Alternatively, telephone 0300 999 5090 to request a pack to be sent.
- Check that the patient, whether they have PMR or GCA or both, is aware of the cardinal signs and symptoms of GCA and the danger of damage to sight if GCA remains untreated.
- Check that the patient is able to pronounce the name of their condition.
- As the patient progresses, ask at regular check-ups whether they feel they need support from other sufferers to help them manage their condition.
- Do give time to discuss tapering strategies with patients, and do not pressurize patients to taper steroids too quickly.

References

1. Kennedy A, Reeves D, Bower P, et al. The effectiveness and cost effectiveness of a national lay-led self care support programme for patients with long-term conditions: a pragmatic randomised controlled trial. *J Epidemiol Community Health* 2007; 61:254–61.

2. Gilbert K. Polly Wotsit and the Giant Dragon: the patient's perspective on PMR and GCA. Second International Symposium and Imaging Workshop Giant Cell Arteritis, Polymyalgia Rheumatica and Large Vessel Vasculitis. *Rheumatology* 2014; 53 Suppl 2:i4–i5.

3. Arthritis Research UK. *Giant Cell Arteritis.* [Patient information booklet] Chesterfield: ARUK, 2011.

4. Arthritis Research UK. *Polymyalgia Rheumatica.* [Patient information booklet] Chesterfield: ARUK, 2014.

5. Gilbert K. *Polymyalgia Rheumatica and Giant Cell Arteritis: A Survival Guide.* London: PMRGCAuk, 2014.

Index

Tables, figures, and boxes are indicated by an italic *t*, *f*, and *b* following the page number.

A

abatacept 101
adalimumab 19,
    91*t*, 93, 98
adhesion molecule
    expression 20
adrenal suppression 129
adventitial vessel
    inflammation 59
AGATA (Abatacept
    in GCA and
    Takayasu's
    arteritis)
    trial 101
alkaline phosphatase
    levels 44
amaurosis fugax 35,
    104, 106
    differential diagnosis 77
anakinra 90*t*, 93, 101
aneurysms 36,
    109–11, 127
angiogenesis
    16–17*f*,18,20
annexin A1 45
anterior ischaemic optic
    neuropathy
    (AION) 35
anticardiolipin
    antibodies 44–5
anticyclic citrullinated
    peptide antibodies
    (ACPAs) 44, 74
antineutrophil cytoplasmic
    antibodies
    (ANCAs) 44
antinuclear antibodies
    (ANAs) 44
antiproteinase-3
    (anti-PR3) 44
aortic involvement 19, 36,
    109–11, 127
    FDG-PET
        findings 64, 65*f*
    magnetic resonance
        imaging 68
Arthritis Care 149*t*
Arthritis Research
    UK 149*t*
arthritis vasculitis,
    exclusion of 43
aspirin, in visual loss 108
atherosclerosis, FDG-PET
    findings 66
autoimmunity 44–5
axillary arteries
    anatomy 54*f*
    imaging 68
    ultrasound 55–6*f*

B

azathioprine 90*t*, 92, 98

B

bacterial endocarditis,
    differential
    diagnosis 76
B cells, role in
    pathogenesis 15
biological agents 90*t*, 93,
    98, 101
biopsy-negative GCA 60
bisphosphonates 114,
    135–6
brain-derived
    neurotrophic
    factor (BDNF) 19
bursitis 20, 27
    FDG-PET
        appearance 30*f*
    magnetic resonance
        imaging 69
    ultrasound
        appearance 50*tf*,
        51*f*

C

calcium, dietary
    intake 113
calcium pyrophosphate
    deposition disease
    (CPPD) 73, 75
calcium supplementation
    135–6
canakinumab 101
cancer
    differentiation
        from PMR 76
    exclusion of 43
cancer risk 7
cardiovascular
    disease risk 7
cardiovascular risk
    factors 6, 136
carotid arteries,
    magnetic
    resonance
    imaging 69
central retinal artery
    occlusion 104*f*
cerebrovascular ischaemic
    events 36
cervical bursitis 69
*Chlamydia
    pneumoniae* 4, 5
ciclosporin 90*t*, 92, 98
classification criteria,
    PMR 29*t*–30

claudication, GCA-related
    34, 135
clinical presentation
    of GCA 33–7, 34*b*, 35*t*
    of PMR 25–7
colour Doppler imaging
    of temporal
        arteritis 53*f*
    pitfalls 54*t*
    use in temporal artery
        biopsy 60
comorbidities 111
    management and
        monitoring 135–6
    socioeconomic
        impact 141–2
connective tissue diseases,
    exclusion of 43
constitutional symptoms
    of GCA 36
    of PMR 26
corticosteroids *see*
    glucocorticoids
cough, GCA-related 37
cranial neuropathies
    37, 106
C-reactive protein
    (CRP) 44, 45
    remission and relapse
        criteria
        in GCA 121
        in PMR 120
creatine kinase 44
crowned dens
    syndrome 75
cyclophosphamide 90*t*,
    92–3, 98
cytokines, role in
    pathogenesis
    13–14, 15, 19, 20

D

dapsone 90*t*, 98
definitions 3
demographics,
    PMR 25
dendritic cells, role in
    pathogenesis 13
diabetes, use of
    FDG-PET 68
diagnosis 134–5
    laboratory
        findings 43–5

magnetic resonance
    imaging 68–9*f*
positron emission
    tomography
    64–8
in prognostic
    studies 126
socioeconomic
    impact 139–40
sources of support
    147, 148–9
ultrasound
    examination
    in large-vessel
        GCA 55–6*f*
    in PMR 49–53
    of the temporal
        artery 53*f*–5
differential diagnosis
    of GCA 76–8
    of PMR 73–6, 74*f*
diplopia 106
direct medical
    costs 140–1*f*
disease activity
    determination
    in GCA 120–1
    imaging
        methods 121–2
    in PMR
        activity
            score 120, 121*b*
        remission and
            relapse criteria
            119–20*b*
disease burden *see*
    socioeconomic
    impact
disease-modifying
    anti-rheumatic
    drugs
    (DMARDs) 90*t*,
    92–3, 98
    see also methotrexate

E

elderly-onset rheumatoid
    arthritis (EORA),
    differential
    diagnosis 73–4
endothelin-1, role in
    pathogenesis 19
enthesitis 27
    FDG-PET
        appearance 30*f*
environmental
    factors 4–5
epidemiology 4–7, 133

151

erythrocyte
   sedimentation rate
   (ESR) 43–4, 45
prognostic
   significance 91t
remission and relapse
   criteria
      in GCA 121
      in PMR 120
etanercept 19, 91t, 93, 98
ethnic differences,
   PMR 25–6
EULAR/ACR classification
   criteria for
   PMR 29t–30
exercise 146

F

FDG-PET see positron
   emission
   tomography
fever, GCA-related 36
fibrinoid necrosis 59
flares
   management 84, 86
      biological
      agents 98, 101
      DMARD therapy 98
   prevention 97–8
fracture risk
   assessment 113,
   114, 136
functional limitations 27

G

gastroprotection 135
gel phenomenon 26–7
gender differences,
   PMR 26, 129
genetic factors 5–6t,
   12–13
genomic effects,
   glucocorticoids
   81, 82f
gevokizumab (GVK) 101
GiACTA RCT 98, 101
giant cell arteritis (GCA)
   association with
   PMR 129
   clinical presentation
   33–7, 34b, 35t
      visual
      symptoms 103–6
   complications 108–11,
   110b, 127
   definition 3
   diagnosis 134–5
      delayed
      recognition 106
      laboratory
      findings 43–5
      in large-vessel
      GCA 55–6f
      magnetic resonance
      imaging 68–9f
      physical
      examination 29
      positron emission
      tomography 63–8
      temporal artery
      biopsy 59–61

temporal artery
   ultrasound 53f–5
differential
   diagnosis 76–8
disease activity
   determination
   120–1
   imaging 121–2
epidemiology 4–7, 133
key points 108b
occult disease 106
outcome
   parameters 122
pathogenesis 11–19
patient
   education 145–50
polymyalgia
   arteritica 100f
prognosis 125–7
socioeconomic
   impact 139–42
treatment
   BSR guidelines 107b
   duration 127–9, 129
   fast-track
   pathway 107f
   flare management
   84, 86
   glucocorticoids
   84–6, 85t
   primary care
   management 135
   relapse and
   refractory
   disease 98–101
   sight loss
   management
   106–8
   steroid-sparing agents
   90–1t, 92–3
glucocorticoids
   adverse effects 111,
   113b, 135
      osteoporosis
      prophylaxis
      113–14
      risk factors for 91t
      socioeconomic
      impact 142
   benefit to risk ratio 86
   duration of treatment
   84, 127–9
   effect on FDG-PET
   findings 67
   effect on TAB
   findings 60
   EULAR
   recommendations
   85t
   long-term
   treatment 128
   mechanisms of
   action 81–3, 82f
   therapeutic regimens
   83–6, 126
      in GCA 135
      in PMR 134
      in relapse
      treatment 84, 86
      tapering therapy 129
      in visual loss 107b–8
   withdrawal
   symptoms 129

H

hallucinations 106
halo sign, temporal
   artery ultrasound
   53f, 121
headache
   differential
   diagnosis 77–8
   GCA-related 33–4
helplines 146–8
hip, ultrasound
   examination
   49–50, 50tf
histopathology
   IFNγ and IL-17A
   expression 14f
   multinucleated giant
   cells 14f
   neovascularization 18f
   temporal artery
   biopsy 12f,
   14f, 59–61
HLA-DRB1*04 5, 6t, 13
Horner syndrome 106
hypothyroidism,
   differentiation
   from PMR 76

I

imaging
   disease activity
   determination
   121–2
   in suspected large vessel
   vasculitis 112f
   see also magnetic
   resonance imaging;
   positron emission
   tomography;
   ultrasound
   examination
imatinib 101
incidence rates 4
   of GCA 5t
   of PMR 6t
infections
   differential
   diagnosis 43, 76
   role in pathogenesis 4
inflammation 11–12f
   amplification
   cascades 15–18
   role of B cells 15
   role of neutrophils 15
   T-cell activation
   and functional
   differentiation
   13–15
inflammatory
   markers 44, 45
   remission and relapse
   criteria
      in GCA 121
      in PMR 120
infliximab 19, 91t, 93, 98
initial treatment
   in GCA 84
   in PMR 83
interferon gamma
   (IFNγ), role in
   pathogenesis
   13, 15

interleukins
   IL-1 blockade 101
   IL-6 15, 16–17f, 18, 20
      serum levels 44,
      45, 121
   IL-6R blockade see
   tocilizumab
   IL-17A 13–14
   IL-17 blockade 101
intravenous pulse
   therapy 84
   mechanisms of
   action 82
ischaemic
   complications 34,
   36, 108–9f, 127

J

jaw claudication 34, 135
joint examination 27
   ultrasound imaging
   49–52

L

laboratory findings 43–5
large-vessel vasculitis
   36, 109–10
   biological therapies 101
   complications 127
   imaging 112f, 121–2
   FDG-PET 68f
   ultrasound 55–6f
leflunomide 90t, 92, 98
lifestyle issues 146

M

macrophages, role in
   pathogenesis
   13, 15, 18
magnetic resonance
   imaging
   (MRI) 68–9f
   disease activity
   determination 122
malignancies
   cancer risk 7
   differentiation
   from PMR 76
   exclusion of 43
matrix metalloproteases
   (MMPs), role
   in pathogenesis 18
methotrexate 98
   in GCA 90t, 92
   in PMR 89, 90t, 91–2
methylprednisolone
   intravenous pulse
   therapy 84
   mechanisms of
   action 82
   in visual loss 108
   see also glucocorticoids
microcrystalline
   arthritis 75
microscopic polyangiitis
   (MPA), differential
   diagnosis 75–6
migraine 78
morning stiffness 26–7

musculoskeletal
symptoms 26–7
association
with GCA 37
mycophenolate
mofetil 90t, 93, 98
Mycoplasma pneumoniae 4

N

neovascularization
16–17f, 18f, 20
nerve growth factor
(NGF) 19
neurological disease,
differential
diagnosis 77–8
neuropeptide
expression 20
neutrophils, role in
pathogenesis 15
non-genomic effects,
glucocorticoids 82f

O

occipital arteries, magnetic
resonance
imaging 69
occult GCA 106
ocular ischaemic
syndrome 106
onset of symptoms, PMR
26
ophthalmoplegia 106
osteoporosis prophylaxis
113–14, 135–6

P

parainfluenza virus 4
parvovirus B19 4, 5
pathogenesis 11–12
amplification cascades
15–18, 16–17f
cardiovascular risk
factors 6
environmental factors
and infectious
agents 4–5
genetic factors 5–6t,
12–13
role of B cells 15
role of neutrophils 15
synovial inflammation
19–20
T-cell activation
and functional
differentiation
13–15
vascular injury 18–19
vascular remodelling
and occlusion 19
patient education
136, 145–6
action checklist 150
helplines 146–8
support groups 148–9
web forums 149–50
Patient UK 149t
pentraxin 3 (PTX3) 45
periadventitial vessel
inflammation 59

peripheral
neuropathies 37
physical examination
in GCA 29, 37
in PMR 27–9
physiotherapy 146
platelet-derived
growth factors
(PDGFs), role
in pathogenesis
18, 19
PMR and GCA Scotland
148, 149t
PMRGCAuk 146–8
involvement in web
forums 149
PMR-GCA UK North East
Support 149t
polymorphisms 13
polymyalgia arteritica 100f
polymyalgia
rheumatica (PMR)
association with
GCA 37,
52–3, 128–9
classification
criteria 29t–30
clinical
presentation 25–7
complications 111
definition 3
diagnosis 134
laboratory
findings 43–5
magnetic resonance
imaging 69
physical
examination 27–9
positron emission
tomography
63–8, 67f, 68f
ultrasound 49–53
differential diagnosis
73–6, 74f
disease activity
determination
imaging 121–2
remission and relapse
criteria 119–20b
epidemiology 4–7, 133
evaluation for GCA 29
gender differences 129
indications for
specialist
review 134b, 135b
outcome
parameters 122
pathogenesis 19–21
patient
education 145–50
prognosis 125–7
socioeconomic
impact 139–42
health services
utilization 140f
treatment
duration 127–9,
128f
glucocorticoids
83–4, 85t, 86
management
algorithm 99f
primary care
management 134

relapse and
refractory
disease 98–101
steroid-sparing
agents 89–93
polymyalgia rheumatica
activity score
(PMR-AS)
120, 121b
polymyositis (PM) 75
positron emission
tomography
(FDG-PET) 63–4,
65f, 110f–11
caveats 66–8
diagnostic
use 64–6, 74, 76
disease activity
determination
121, 122
in PMR 30f
posterior ischaemic
optic neuropathy
(PION) 35
prednisolone
in GCA 84
in PMR 83
see also glucocorticoids
primary care
diagnosis
of GCA 134–5
of PMR 134
epidemiology 133
management
of comorbidities
135–6
of GCA 135
of PMR 134
patient education and
counselling 136
prognosis
general considerations
125–6
optimization 126
outcome studies 7
prolonged therapy,
risk factors
for 91t
proteinuria 44
proximal symptoms 26–7
PTPN22 (protein tyrosine
phosphatase,
non-receptor type
22) 5–6
puffy oedematous hand
syndrome (RS3PE
syndrome)
27–8f, 37, 75

R

refractory disease
biological therapies 98,
101
DMARD therapy 98
relapse 128
biological
therapies 98, 101
DMARD therapy 98
gender differences 129
glucocorticoid
therapy 84, 86
risk factors for 91t
relapse criteria, PMR 120b

remission criteria, PMR
119–20b
research
on biological agents 93
on DMARDs 90–1t,
92–3
outcome studies 7
into pathogenesis
4–6, 12–13
rheumatoid arthritis 30
differentiation from
PMR 73–4
FDG-PET findings 66
ultrasound findings 52f
rheumatoid factor 44, 74
risk factors
for glucocorticoid-related
adverse effects 83,
85t, 86, 91t, 113b
for ischaemic
complications
6, 44
for relapse 91t
risk stratification 97–8
rituximab 90t, 93, 101
RS3PE (remitting
seronegative
symmetrical
synovitis with
pitting oedema)
syndrome
27–8f, 37, 75

S

scalp necrosis 109f
secukinumab 101
shoulder, ultrasound
examination
in PMR 49–50, 50tf
in rheumatoid
arthritis 52f
sleep disturbance 27
socioeconomic impact
direct medical
costs 141f
establishing a
diagnosis 139–40
health services
utilization 140f
management of
late-stage disease
and complications
141–2
treatment of active
disease 140–1
specialist referral
in GCA 135
in PMR 134b, 135b
spondyloarthropathies,
differential
diagnosis 75
statins 7
steroids see
glucocorticoids
steroid-sparing
agents 90–1t, 98
biological agents 93
methotrexate 89–92
non-methotrexate
DMARDs 92–3
stroke, risk in larger
vessel
vasculitis 109

subarachnoid
    haemorrhage
        77–8
subclavian artery
    involvement
        FDG-PET
            findings 63–4, 65f
        magnetic resonance
            imaging 69f
support groups
    146, 148–9
synovial inflammation
    imaging 28f
        MRI 69
        ultrasound 27
    pathogenesis 19–20

T

TABUL (Temporal Artery
    Biopsy versus
    Ultrasound)
    study 55
Takayasu's arteritis
    (TAK), differential
    diagnosis 78
tapering regimens 129
    in GCA 84, 108
    in PMR 83–4
T cells
    activation and functional
        differentiation
        13–15
    role in PMR 20
temporal arteries
    anatomy 54f
    magnetic resonance
        imaging 69
temporal artery biopsy
    (TAB) 12f

biopsy-negative GCA
    60
    effect of glucocorticoid
        therapy 60–1
    histopathology 59–60
    sample size and
        location 60
temporal artery
    ultrasound 53f–5
    pitfalls 54t
    in PMR 52–3
tenosynovitis
    magnetic resonance
        imaging 69
    ultrasound appearance
        50tf, 51f
thyroid disease, differential
    diagnosis 76
TNF blocking agents 19
    see also adalimumab;
        etanercept;
        infliximab
tocilizumab (TCZ) 19,
    90t, 93, 98
toll-like receptors
    (TLRs), role in
    pathogenesis 13
tonic pupil 106
transactivation and
    transrepression,
    glucocorticoids 81
transforming growth
    factor beta
    (TGFβ), role in
    pathogenesis
    13, 19
treatment
    EULAR
        recommendations
        97–8
    glucocorticoids 81–4

adverse effects 111,
    113b–14
benefit to risk
    ratio 86
duration of use 84
EULAR
    recommendations
    85t
in relapse 84, 86
socioeconomic
    impact 140–2
steroid-sparing
    agents 90–1t, 98
    biological agents 93
    methotrexate 89–92
    non-methotrexate
        DMARDs 92–3
tumour necrosis factor
    alpha (TNFα)
    role in pathogenesis 12,
        16–17f, 18, 19
    TNFα blockers
        91t, 93, 98

U

ultrasound examination
    disease activity
        determination 121
    in large-vessel
        GCA 55–6f
    in PMR 28f, 30, 49–53
    in temporal
        arteritis 53–5
    in temporal artery
        biopsy 60

V

varicella zoster virus 5

vascular endothelial
    growth factor
    (VEGF)
    expression 20
vascular injury,
    pathogenesis
    18–19
vascular remodelling 19
vascular stenosis 127
vasculitis
    differential
        diagnosis 75–6, 78
    ultrasound
        examination 55–6f
    see also giant cell
        arteritis; large
        vessel vasculitis
Vasculitis UK 149t
visual symptoms
    34–5, 103–6
    differential diagnosis 77
    fluorescein
        angiography 105f
    management
        106–8, 135
        fast-track
            pathway 107f
    risk factors for 106
    socioeconomic
        impact 141–2
vitamin D
    supplementation
    113, 135–6
voluntary
    organizations 149t
    PMRGCAuk 146–8
    support groups 148–9

W

web forums 149–50